Ritalin-Free Kids

ALSO BY THE AUTHORS

Prozac-Free
Rage-Free Kids
Homeopathic Self-Care
Whole Woman Homeopathy
The Patient's Guide to Homeopathic Medicine

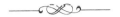

Ritalin-Free Kids

Safe and Effective Homeopathic
Medicine for ADHD and Other
Behavioral and Learning Problems

REVISED 2ND EDITION

Judyth Reichenberg-Ullman,
N.D., M.S.W.

Robert Ullman, N.D.

PRIMA PUBLISHING

Published by Prima Publishing, Roseville, California. Member of the Crown
Publishing Group, a division of Random House, Inc.

Random House, Inc. New York, Toronto, London, Sydney, Auckland

PRIMA PUBLISHING and colophon are trademarks of Random House, Inc.,
registered with the United States Patent and Trademark Office.

This book is intended for educational purposes only. It is not intended to
diagnose, treat, give medical advice for a specific condition, or in any way
replace the services of a qualified medical practitioner. Readers are advised
to consult a qualified medical practitioner before treating any specific condition. The publisher and the authors therefore disclaim any responsibility for
any injury or damage suffered from the use of any information contained
herein.

When making general references to patients, the authors alternate between
"he" and "she" for the purpose of equality of gender reference. The cases in
this book are true stories from the authors' clinical practice. They have tried
as much as possible to use the words of the patients and to tell their stories
as they were told to them. The authors have changed the names to protect
confidentiality.

Library of Congress Cataloging-in-Publication Data

Reichenberg-Ullman, Judyth.
   Ritalin-free kids : safe and effective homeopathic medicine for ADHD and
other behavioral and learning problems / Judyth Reichenberg-Ullman,
Robert Ullman.—2nd ed., rev.
      p. cm.
   Includes bibliographical references and index.
   ISBN 0-7615-2769-9
   1. Attention-deficit hyperactivity disorder—Homeopathic treatment. 2.
Attention-deficit hyperactivity disorder—Chemotherapy—Complications. 3.
Methylphenidate hydrochloride—Side effects. I. Ullman, Robert. II. Title.
RX531.A77 U45 2000
618.92'858906—dc21   00-062356

01 02 03 HH 10 9 8 7 6 5 4 3 2
Printed in the United States of America
Second Edition

Visit us online at www.primapublishing.com

———∞———

Contents

Foreword by Edward Hallowell, M.D.   ix
Preface by Edward H. Chapman, M.D., D.Ht.   xiii
Acknowledgments   xvi
Introduction   xvii

PART ONE
The Conventional View of ADHD

1. **Drifty, Driven, and Daring**
   The Typical Characteristics of ADHD   3

2. **Life in Overdrive**
   Growing Up with ADHD   10

3. **Epidemic or Overdiagnosis?**
   Can So Many Children Have ADHD?   22

4. **The ADHD Pressure Cooker**
   Kids, Teachers, Parents, and Doctors
   All Feel the Heat   33

5. **To Drug or Not to Drug**
   The Pros and Cons of Conventional Treatment
   for ADHD and Other Behavioral
   and Mood Disorders   41

6. **Different Strokes for Different Folks**
   What Parents and Kids Say
   About Drugs for ADHD   60

PART TWO
Homeopathy: A Whole Child Approach

7. All About Homeopathy
Natural Medicine That Works   71

8. A Better Answer Than Ritalin
Homeopathy Is a Highly Effective
Treatment for ADHD   82

9. Unique Treatment for Unique Individuals
Treating People, Not Diagnoses   95

10. Changing Children's Lives with Homeopathy
What Parents Say About
Homeopathic Treatment   101

11. Living with and Learning from a Child
with ADHD
Tips for Parents   108

PART THREE
**Real Stories of Real People: Successful
Homeopathic Treatment of ADHD**

12. Kids on the Move
Attention Deficit with Hyperactivity   117

13. "I Have to Tell Him Everything Ten Times"
Attention Deficit Without Hyperactivity   129

14. "You Never Know What She's Up To"
Sneaky, Mischievous Kids   144

15. "If I Say Black, He Says White"
Oppositional, Defiant Behavior   153

16. "I'm Gonna Chop Off His Head "
ADHD with Violence and Rage   166

17. "Won't I Ever Outgrow This?"
Adults with ADHD   188

PART FOUR
**Homeopathic Treatment of Learning
Disabilities, the Autism Spectrum, and
Other Mental and Emotional Problems**

18. Enhancing the Learning Curve
Through Homeopathy
Learning Disabilities
and Developmental Delays   209

19. A Terrifying World
Fearful, Anxious Kids   230

20. "I Feel Bad About Myself. I Have No Friends."
Depressed Kids   250

PART FIVE
**Expanding Your Knowledge
of Homeopathy**

21. The Most Commonly Asked Questions About
Homeopathic Treatment for ADHD   267

22. Our Society Needs Homeopathy Now   275

Appendix: Learning More   279
Glossary   284
Index   290
About the Authors   295

*To our parents, who raised us with love,
support, and guidance and instilled in us
the confidence to pursue our dreams
and aspirations*

*To the many children whom we have
enjoyed seeing as patients,
some of whose stories appear in this book*

*To their parents for having the open-mindedness
and trust to seek out homeopathy*

*To other children suffering from physical,
emotional, behavioral, or learning problems—
may homeopathy offer you and your parents
a new ray of hope*

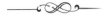

Foreword

When Judyth Reichenberg-Ullman and Robert Ullman sent me this book, the first thing I noticed was how impossible it would be for me to spell their names. How could I write a foreword to a book if I couldn't get past the spelling of the authors' names? But I reminded myself that one of the precepts I try to live by is never to shy away from the unfamiliar, so I tackled the names and learned how to spell them (I hope!).

The second thing I noticed was that this was a book that had Ritalin in its title. Usually such books attack the use of Ritalin and other stimulant medications. Since I am an expert on the treatment of ADHD, and since I do prescribe stimulant medication for some of my patients, it seemed odd that the authors would ask me to write an endorsement for a book that I imagined attacked what I do in my practice. But, once again, I reminded myself of my precept not to shy away from the unfamiliar. So I read the book.

I am very glad I did.

This book taught me a great deal. Before reading it, I knew almost nothing about homeopathic medicine. This book opened my eyes. Now I know some of the basics, and I want to learn even more. I even want to look into the possibility of finding a homeopathic physician to join my practice.

I will continue to recommend, as my first-line choice, the use of stimulant medication to treat ADHD. The track record of these medications is superb. Ritalin and other similar medications, such as Adderal and Dexedrine, have changed millions of lives dramatically for the better, in both children and adults. I know this because I have seen it up close in my practice for years. I know that these medications work and that they work well. I also know that they are very safe as long as they are used under proper medical supervision.

However, stimulant medications are not for everyone. About 20 to 30 percent of children and adults with ADHD will not respond well to stimulant medication, so they need an alternative. Also, many people, for good and not-so-good reasons, refuse even to consider taking stimulant medication because of all the bad reports they have heard about them. These people also need an alternative.

Ritalin-Free Kids provides such an alternative. This book will really open your eyes to the possibility of homeopathic medicine, not only for treating ADHD, but also for treating a number of emotional and learning problems, as well as some behavioral problems like anger outbursts and bedwetting.

It is not hocus-pocus. Homeopaths have produced a respectable scientific literature that deserves greater public and professional attention. I hope this book will help the field gain such attention.

Beyond that, I hope this book will help open people's minds to the possibility of seeking help from a homeopathic physician.

Drs. Reichenberg-Ullman and Ullman have written a clear, balanced, and persuasive book. They are not polemicists, and they do not want to run down conventional medicine or its practitioners. They simply want to offer their own valuable experience as clinicians and to call attention to the research in their field.

I believe they have done an excellent job.

Edward Hallowell, M.D.,
Coauthor of *Driven to Distraction*
and author of *Worry* and *Connect*

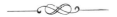

Preface

In some schools, as many as 30 percent of the children are on Ritalin. Does this epidemic of attention deficit/hyperactivity disorder reflect something new? Are we just diagnosing better? Are the latent weaknesses of the human nervous system becoming overwhelmed by the pace and complexity of life in the information age? No one has enough time. We are flooded with sound and video bites. There is more to do than anyone has time for. Kids don't have time or space to be kids. The expectations are enormous. Each of us can experience how our nervous systems are overflowing with the stress this environment creates. Although there are similarities among people's strategies, each of us has our own unique way of coping and adapting.

People with ADHD manifest their distress differently depending on their unique constitutions. Many are over-stimulated, distracted, and restless. Others become hyper-vigilant, withdrawn, and compulsive. Others act out, become disruptive or aggressive. All have trouble with self-esteem in their struggle to function. All these various presentations might be labeled ADHD. Despite the diversity, the conventional approach boils the problem down into a single diagnosis, which is typically treated by a single class of drugs. As long as medications are continued, the symptoms are somewhat controlled, much to the relief of the child or adult, teachers, and parents. Few patients ever outgrow their need for drug therapy. Many stop because of the side effects, limited effectiveness, or to try something different.

Before you give your child stimulants, read this book. *Ritalin-Free Kids* describes another approach—one that respects and takes advantage of the diversity of people with symptoms of ADHD; an approach that stimulates the unique adaptive mechanisms each person carries within. Homeopathy is a system of medicine that is highly individualized and can help people move toward optimal health. The case examples in this book demonstrate that, when used alone or as a complement to conventional therapies, homeopathic medicines can improve the function of people with ADHD to the point where conventional medicines are often no longer necessary.

The authors describe their experience gained from treating more than 1,500 children and adults with behavioral and learning problems. The words of the patients tell the story. Positive evidence is accumulating from clinical and laboratory studies to support the claims of homeopathy. Much more rigorous research is needed into the homeopathic approach before it gains wider acceptance. The clinical experience described in this book will undoubtedly catch the eye of those who have the resources to devote to scientific inquiry. The goal of medical research is to bring safe and effective therapies to the public. The evidence provided by these two pioneering practitioners will undoubtedly stimulate the dialogue between conventional and complementary health care providers, to the benefit of both.

For those who need support in their struggle with ADHD and can't wait for the years of research, they can be assured from two hundred years experience using homeopathic medicines that they are safe. Make your own judgments about effectiveness based on the patients' stories presented. Your conventional doctor may be skeptical if you choose to use homeopathy. Don't let that stop you, or stop you from telling him or her. Your doctor will then have the chance to grow with you. But take the advice of the authors and seek assistance from well-trained homeopathic providers who are willing to work with you and your doctors. Then everyone stands to learn and benefit.

Edward H. Chapman, M.D., D.Ht.
Past President, American Institute of Homeopathy
Clinical Instructor, Harvard University
     School of Medicine

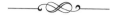

Acknowledgments

We thank Edward Hallowell, M.D., for taking time out of a busy schedule to write the enjoyable and encouraging foreword of our revised edition; Ted Chapman, M.D., for his articulate preface; Shane McCamey and Miranda Castro for heartily encouraging us to write this book; Leslie Howle, who is responsible for Prima first learning about our work; and Susan Silva and Tara Mead, both of whom have made the editing process relatively pleasurable and painless. We also thank Jennifer Jacobs, M.D., M.P.H., Richard Solomon, M.D., and Dana Ullman, M.P.H., for generously offering their time to review our book. We are especially grateful to Rajan Sankaran, Divya Chhabra Jayesh Shah, Nandita Shah, Sujit Chatterjee, Sunil Anand, and Sudhir Baldhota for enlivening our practice of homeopathy and enhancing our ability to use this wonderful form of medicine to help many patients.

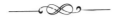

Introduction

Attention deficit/hyperactivity disorder (ADHD), the most common behavioral disorder in children, is being diagnosed in epidemic proportions. Of these youngsters, 65 to 75 percent are being given prescriptions for stimulant medications.[1] At the time we wrote the first edition of *Ritalin-Free Kids* in 1996, at least two million children in the United States were taking stimulant medications (primarily Ritalin, Dexedrine, and Cylert) for ADHD. That is more than one in every thirty children ages five to eighteen. In 1988 half a million children were prescribed stimulants for ADHD. The number quadrupled in only eight years. Physicians in this country prescribe five times the quantity of stimulants for children as the rest of the countries of the world combined. These are regulated by the Drug Enforcement Agency (DEA).[2] A report by the United Nations in 1996 revealed that 3 to 5 percent of all schoolchildren in the

---

[1] Linda Robison, David Sclar, Tracy Skaer, and Richard Galin, "National Trends in the Prevalence of Attention-Deficit/Hyperactivity Disorder and the Prescribing of Methylphenidate Among School-age Children: 1990–1995." *Clinical Pediatrics* 38: 216 (1999).

[2] The Merrow Report, *ADD—A Dubious Diagnosis.* Public Broadcasting System. October 20, 1994.

United States were taking Ritalin.[3] In 1990, the number of children diagnosed with ADHD was 750,000. By 1996 the figure approached four million. The DEA documented the production of Ritalin to have increased by nearly 500 percent from 1991 to 1996 and from less than 2,000 kilograms in 1986 to 9,000 kilograms in 1995.[4] Ninety percent of the Ritalin produced in the United States is used within this country,[5] and 90 percent of children with ADHD in the United States who are on medications take Ritalin.[6] The number of physcian office-based visits of children presenting with a diagnosis of ADHD increased two and a half times from 1990 to 1995.[7] The diagnosis of ADHD in adults increased sevenfold from 1985 to 1994.[8]

Ritalin is also known to be a fairly common street drug. The Drug Abuse Warning Network data on emergency room visits indicated a sixfold increase in patients who admitted to taking Ritalin from 1990 to 1995.[9] The DEA has received reports of thefts of Ritalin, street sales, drug rings, illegal importation into the United States

---

[3] "Misuse of Ritalin by Schoolchildren Prompts Warning," *Seattle Times,* March 27, 1996.

[4] Larry Goldman, Myron Genel, Rebecca Bezman, and Alan, "Diagnosis and Treatment of Attention-Deficit/Hyperactivity Disorder in Children and Adolescents." *Journal of the American Medical Association* 279(14): 1104 (1988).

[5] Ibid., 1104.

[6] Ibid., 1105.

[7] Robison *et al.,* 209.

[8] Edmund Higgins, "A Comparative Analysis of Antidepressants and Stimulants for the Treatment of Adults with Attention-deficit Hyperactivity Disorder." *The Journal of Family Practice* 48(1): 15–20 (1999).

[9] Goldman *et al.,* 1104.

from other countries, and illegal sales by health professionals, as well as theft of school supplies of Ritalin.[10]

Even more alarming is the "off label" dispensing of stimulants and antidepressants to youngsters under the age of six. Not only is there inadequate research on the effectiveness of these drugs in children who may be barely past toddlerhood, but there are no data on the long-term effects of psychotropic drugs on brain development. Dr. Joseph Coyle, chair of Harvard Medical School's Department of Psychiatry, warns that "The period between birth and four is a time of tremendous change in the maturation of the brain. . . . We need to be very cautious."[11]

Imagine the following scenario: your eight-year-old son, Jesse, has just entered second grade. Within three weeks of starting the school year, you receive a note from his new teacher. She has observed that Jesse wriggles around in his seat entirely too much and has a hard time keeping his hands off of the children around him. She finds his repetitive questions annoying and disruptive. Jesse appears to tune out much of the time in class, and when it's time to write down the homework assignments, he's out in left field. His handwriting is a disaster. You give the teacher a call and assure her that Jesse simply needs more time to adjust. You're aware that he's a high-spirited child, but he'll be okay.

Within two months, the teacher calls you in for a conference. You enter the room, with a sinking feeling, waiting for the shoe to drop. If Jesse is really over the top or the school district is particularly strict, the counselor and even the principal and psychologist may have

---

[10] Goldman *et al.,* 1104.

[11] Claudia Kalb, "Drugged-out Toddlers." *Newsweek,* March 6, 2000, 53.

been called to attend the meeting as well. "Have you heard of ADHD?" she (or they) asks. "Have you thought of putting your child on Ritalin?" In some cases, you may even be warned that Jesse cannot remain in the classroom unless he is medicated. You sulk out of the room, bewildered, or you are seething with anger at having been set up, or you are really ticked off with Jesse for letting himself, and you, down or you blame yourself for being an inadequate parent. Or all of the above.

Is it legal for a teacher to tell you that your child has ADHD? Probably not, since she is not a doctor. Does she have the right to tell you that he can't stay in her classroom unless he is medicated? Probably not. But in our experience, this happens to a number of parents every day. Many of them end up, with their children, in the office of their family physician, a psychologist, or a psychiatrist, seeking prescriptions for amphetamines for their children. Other parents initially refuse to consider giving drugs to their children, then change their minds out of fear that they will ruin their children's opportunities to learn and mature normally. Once children like Jesse begin taking stimulants, they often need to continue the medication for five to ten years, sometimes for life. There is yet another route at least several thousand parents have taken, thanks in large part to their interest in *Ritalin-Free Kids,* which has made it into the hands of over 50,000 readers. That is homeopathic medicine. It is these parents (and adults) who find themselves, instead, sitting in the office of a homeopath.

We offer you an alternative to Ritalin and other stimulant medications. If you or your child has been diagnosed with ADHD and you are looking for non-drug alternative, BEFORE YOU FILL THAT PRESCRIPTION FOR STIMULANTS, READ THIS BOOK! Homeopathic medicine is a safe, effective, and natural treatment for ADHD and an approach that may be entirely new to you and your family (see chapter 7). If you are inspired by this book, which is our hope, please find an experienced homeopath to treat you or your child. DO NOT USE THE INFORMATION IN THIS BOOK TO PRESCRIBE FOR YOUR CHILD'S OR YOUR OWN ADHD. Homeopathic prescribing is an art as well as a science. The success and long-lasting results about which you read in this book and that you may be seeking are only possible under the care of a qualified homeopathic practitioner.

We began treating children with ADHD thirteen years ago. We have been astounded at how significantly, and often dramatically, homeopathy has transformed the lives of many of these children in a very positive way. Jimmy was one of the first children with ADHD whom we treated homeopathically. Here is his story:

Jimmy was a nine-year-old child diagnosed with ADHD. His parents, both in their fifties, had been in and out of alcoholism treatment programs. Jimmy and his younger sister had been shuffled from one foster home to another. Both children had been beaten repeatedly and subjected to profound neglect. In fact, Jimmy was afraid to go into the bathroom because his mother used to beat him there. When Jimmy arrived at the home of the foster mother who brought him to see us, he was filthy. He had not had a haircut for a year. His shoes were three-and-a-half sizes too small.

Jimmy's behavior was extreme. He was active and busy all the time. Due to his disruptive classroom behavior, he had been placed in special-education classes. He jumped up and down constantly, pestered the other children, and exasperated his teacher to such an extent that she insisted Jimmy's foster mother come to school and sit with him in class all day, or he could not attend. And so, devoted as she was to Jimmy's well-being, she did.

This youngster hummed, twiddled, sang, and talked incessantly. He shook rattles, squeezed horns, and grabbed anything he could find to keep himself busy. Jimmy was always moving some part of his body. His hands fidgeted and he swung his legs restlessly. At bedtime, Jumping Jimmy leapt off the bed and prattled to his foster sister even after she had fallen asleep. When Jimmy finally did fall asleep, he tossed and turned all night.

Impatient and impulsive, if Jimmy went out in public with his mom, he wandered away. Despite his uncontrollable restlessness, Jimmy was kind, considerate, and would be the first to give away his candy bar if another child did not have one.

We prescribed for Jimmy the homeopathic medicine *Veratrum album* (white hellebore). Within two days after the medication, his hyperactivity had improved dramatically. Jimmy's teacher called his foster mother to ask what she had done with him. She could take him shopping now and he no longer wandered off. He stopped humming and talking all the time and no longer chattered to his sister after she was asleep. We were able to follow Jimmy's progress for two more years, and he continued to do very well.

Because of the impressive results in Jimmy's case and several others, we began to use homeopathy with many children with ADHD and other behavioral and learning problems. As we wrote articles about our successful cases, parents called us from all over the United States and abroad, asking us to treat their children. We have treated nearly 2,000 children diagnosed with ADHD and other behavioral and learning problems, as well as a number of adults. We include many cases in our book so that you can see for yourself how effective homeopathy is with these children. We estimate our success rate to be 70 percent when the patients continue with homeopathic treatment for at least one year. Kids with ADHD are some of our favorite patients. They can be lively, engaging, bright, entertaining, and witty. However, their extreme behaviors and tendencies can also get them into lots of trouble. Treating these kids, and often their parents or siblings, has become an extremely rewarding aspect of our practice. In many cases, we have found homeopathy to literally turn around their lives.

This book may be your first exposure to homeopathic medicine. As you read on, you will see that prescribing homeopathic medicines for ADHD is a complex, but highly effective and rewarding, process. If you are looking for an alternative to stimulants, you may have found it in this book. Whether or not homeopathy is for you, we sincerely hope that you and your children find health and happiness.

PART ONE

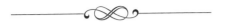

The Conventional View of ADHD

1

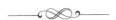

Drifty, Driven, and Daring
The Typical Characteristics of ADHD

Calling Planet Earth . . . Do You Read Me?

ADHD is really more a collection of common features than one discrete group of symptoms that is inevitably present in each child (or adult) thought to have the condition. The consistent factor among those who can legitimately be diagnosed with ADHD is that their problems with attention, hyperactivity, and impulsive behaviors are significant enough to interfere with normal functioning at home, school, or work. Children with ADHD do not all manifest the condition in the same way. Some are dreamy, drifty, or spaced-out, but not hyperactive. They seem lost in the clouds, barely on the planet, and oblivious to most of what occurs around them. Other youngsters seem to be in constant motion, bouncing off the walls, driven, and motorized. Still others cannot wait, interrupt constantly, must be first, and are always seeking out something new or stimulating. This craving is readily satisfied in our sound-bite-a-minute society.

Kids with ADHD have difficulty concentrating and paying attention, especially in situations where they are forced to sit still, such as at school or at their desks at work. At the same time, if the activity is of their own

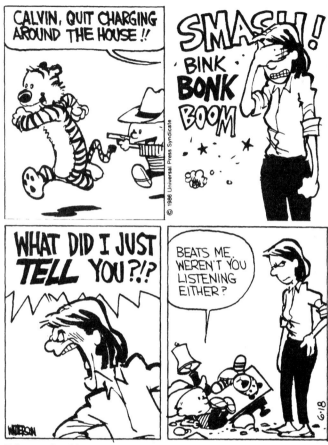

Calvin and Hobbes © (1986) Watterson. Distributed by Universal Press
Syndicate. Reprinted with permission. All rights reserved.

choosing, they may sit for hours, fully engaged in Nintendo, hyperfocused on Pokémon, or 100 percent absorbed in Harry Potter's latest adventures. When they are required to brush their teeth, however, or turn in a homework assignment, take out the garbage, or get dressed for school, they may find it almost impossible to concentrate for more than a few seconds or minutes when so many other, more attractive stimuli vie for their attention.

Tasks at home and at school tend to be done in a hasty, sloppy, and careless fashion and fraught with mistakes. A child or adolescent with ADHD may find it extremely challenging to listen to or write down instructions, start a project without being distracted or procrastinating, and follow through until the task is complete. It is not that he does not *want* to finish what he starts. He just never quite gets around to it. Even if he actually completes a task, he may have been unable to do so within the allotted time. This tendency becomes worse as the child grows up. Many tasks are started, but few are ever finished.

Where DID I Put That Homework Assignment?

The workspace or bedroom of a child with ADHD may look like a candidate for disaster relief. The remains of countless unfinished projects, stacks of papers, or any variety of objects are in utter disarray. Youngsters with attention problems misplace books, homework assignments, jackets, shoes, or their allowance, while their adult counterparts often cannot find car keys, checkbooks, wallets, or those forms they needed to mail to the Internal Revenue Service three weeks earlier. They insist that the objects in question are "in that pile," "around here somewhere," or "under that pizza box over there." Despite their best intentions, they may be careless, clumsy, and accident-prone.

In social situations, folks with ADHD often miss the subtle cues of facial expression, tone of voice, and body language that are central to communication. Their attention may be so limited that they drift off and totally miss what the other person is saying, or fade in and out, only getting enough to embarrass themselves when they try to respond to the conversation they have barely heard. ADHD causes people to have trouble making and keeping friends. As they become older, they forget appointments, dates, and birthdays, or show up late with a lame apology, to the disappointment and dismay of others who were waiting for or depending upon them.

Wired for Sound

When hyperactivity is predominant, a situation more common with children than adults with ADHD, the child may be "wired." Such kids commonly burn off their over-the-top excesses of energy by running back and forth or in circles through the house or by climbing furniture, trees, and even walls. They often engage routinely in reckless activities that terrify their parents, such as riding handlebars, scaling precarious structures, or darting onto a busy street, oblivious to traffic. Some merely wander off, sending parents, or even the police, frantically hunting for them. All children do *some* of these things *some of the time,* but the ADHD child is apt to do them constantly, requiring around-the-clock vigilance and driving their parents to tears, exhaustion, and desperation. We often hear "She never stops going, morning, noon, and night," or "You can turn her on, but you can't turn her off!" Restless squirming, fidgeting with objects, tapping fingers and feet, drumming, and pacing are all ways for a youngster with ADHD to unconsciously mark time and release pent-up nervous energy.

Act First, Think Later

Impulsivity is another major feature of the ADHD picture. Patience is not a virtue common to these children. They refuse to wait for their turns, dash to the head of the line, and throw caution to the wind, acting first and thinking later, usually after something is inadvertently broken, someone is hurt, or it is too late to make the right choice. They may consider instructions irrelevant, or only half hear them. Children with ADHD can be uncomfortably intrusive, interrupting others to blurt out often-inappropriate responses or to make sure their needs are attended to immediately. Children who fit the impulsive picture of ADHD are often described as loud, silly, immature, and incessant talkers. Even when repeatedly reprimanded, they can't seem to bring their behavior into a level of social acceptability. They push and shove to get what they want, grab things from their parents or peers, and go after their desired object or goal with little regard for who or what might be around them.

Intelligent Underachievers

All of these characteristics, depending on the age, the context, and the intensity of expression, can, and frequently do, cause significant problems. These children are singled out in school as troublemakers, clowns, instigators, space cadets, and intelligent underachievers who never work up to their potential. Children with ADHD may be quite bright, even precocious, but cannot seem to succeed in any task that requires sitting still and paying attention, or in applying focused concentration on any task that does not capture their interest. They lose assignments, fail tests, and forget what they were supposed to bring to school or take home. Their grades almost never reflect their true capabilities. ADHD children do much better in small groups or in one-on-one situations. These kids thrive on external structure, being unable to organize their own time or activities, but also chafe under too close or severe a discipline. Easily bored, these individuals constantly seek something novel and may be highly imaginative and inventive. Some children with attention problems, on the other hand, have mild to severe learning disabilities that can worsen their already less-than-stellar school performance.

How Many Times Do I Have to Tell You to Clean Your Room?

At home, parents complain of having to repeat instructions over and over. Children fail to follow through consistently on the simplest chores, being so easily distracted that they completely forget whatever they were told to do moments before. When getting dressed or eating, they take what seems like forever. These youngsters may simply wander off with the task undone or may try to perform three tasks at once, handling none of them well. They need extremely close supervision to get anything done. If punished or reprimanded, either they fall apart, or the effect is very short-lived. Consequences and past experience are blown out of proportion or forgotten. Tantrumming as a way to avoid undesirable or unpleasant tasks may be an artful avoidance strategy for some children with ADHD. Kids like these may want very much to pay attention or to do a good job; they just can't.

The Upside of ADHD

On the positive side, many children with ADHD are bright and eager to please. They can be charming, spontaneous, and fun, with a fresh moment-to-moment approach to life. People often find them more entertaining than irritating when taken in small doses. Creativity runs high in kids and adults with ADHD, and they often have more ideas than they can carry out effectively. They may be artistically gifted and quite sensitive. These youngsters look for the new and interesting challenges of life and can be way ahead of their parents in IQ, innovative thinking, and originality, not to mention computer skills. Individuals with ADHD may be risk takers—if they can avoid breaking bones, they can make breakthroughs that are beyond the reach of the less daring. Or they may be dreamers whose visions can turn into a very gratifying and lucrative reality if they team up with others who are more grounded and follow through on their ideas. If they are provided with an open-ended, flexible environment with enough structure and encouragement to allow follow-through, adults with ADHD can live exciting and fulfilling lives. Some of these individuals do fine without interventions of any kind; others' odds for enjoying and succeeding in life are greatly enhanced with an effective form of help, whether conventional or alternative.

2

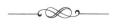

Life in Overdrive
Growing Up with ADHD

Rug Rats on the Run

In our experience, some children can give hints of future ADHD characteristics as early as infancy, or even in the womb. We have found that the following symptoms raise a red flag when a child displays them more frequently or intensely than does the average child.

Restlessness   Infants squirm, kick, and move constantly. They demand to be held, put down, then picked up again. They roll about in their cribs, make every attempt to escape, and crawl around vigorously as soon as they possibly can.

Poor eye contact   Eyes dart about, unable to focus on any one object for very long. Babies may not attend to social cues like smiling or frowning and seem to be in a world of their own.

Sleeplessness   ADHD infants may be very challenging to put to sleep, and they may wake up unusually frequently, to the distress of their weary, sleep-deprived parents. These babies may seem genuinely overamped, over-flowing with energy that simply can't be easily quelled.

Frequent fussiness   Difficult to satisfy, these children often are extraordinarily fussy, demanding ongoing attention and stimulation, while other children are more easily pacified. Whether they are tantrumming or teething, they seem intense. They refuse whatever is offered and are generally disagreeable and hard to please.

Motorized Toddlers

Experts claim that we can identify 60 to 70 percent of ADHD children by age two to three.[1] Parents often tell us that their ADHD toddlers ran before they walked. The traits they have as infants generally intensify as they become more mobile and expressive.

Toddlers on the go   These kids are notorious for reaching tall cabinets and counters in a single bound, leaping over furniture, or hiding in bushes or clothes racks until their parents are beside themselves. They outlast the Energizer bunny and toddle faster than a speeding Hot Wheels.

Need for constant stimulation   You must literally stay at least one step ahead of these little roadrunners to keep them occupied. Whether it is a brand-new Disney video, a trip to the Discovery Zone, or their favorite treat, they are forever looking for the next adventure or gratification.

[1] Thomas Phelan, Ph.D., Lecture, Tukwila, WA, 1/26/96

Reckless, impulsive, and accident-prone   Boys with ADHD have this trait more often than girls. One child, at three, crawled out on the roof through an open bedroom window. Fortunately, his frantic mom reached him before he tumbled off the eaves. Another of our young patients was so daring that he was rushed to the hospital twice in one day, both times for stitches in his head.

Tantrums   All children have tantrums sometimes, but many of our patients erupt multiple times in a single day. These are full-blown tantrums, complete with kicking, biting, pounding, screaming, flailing, and beating their heads on the floor or the nearest wall. Parents find such episodes exhausting, embarrassing, and discouraging.

No need for naps and hard to put to bed   The only respite for many parents is the afternoon nap and when the child is finally put to bed. Unfortunately, these children are often not interested in sleep. There are so many other exciting things to see, do, and experience. It is a matter of who gets worn down the fastest, and there is generally no contest.

Hurting animals   Animals can also fall prey to the overly rambunctious play of ADHD children. This is typically not due to deliberate cruelty, but is more a matter of impulsivity, not paying attention, and lack of judgment. The smaller the animal, the greater the risk that the child will injure it, sometimes fatally.

Pesky Preschoolers

By the time your child is three to five years old, the seeds of ADHD have germinated and begun to sprout.

Watch for the following behaviors to surface at home, at preschool, with the babysitter, and at family and social events.

Defiance and tantrums   All children say "no" and act out in public. With ADHD children, however, the behavior can be extreme and relentless. Parents become embarrassed about even taking their child to the grocery store for fear of a kicking, screaming battle over an ardently desired treat.

Difficulty getting along with peers   ADHD children can lag behind in social skills because they rarely notice the subtle cues that define interactions among children. While other kids are learning to play together and share, these children may alienate others unintentionally with their annoying, bossy, or self-centered behaviors, causing heartbreak for both parents and child alike.

Violence and destruction   Venting frustration and anger leads children to express violence by breaking their own toys or those of other children, damaging their home, their parents' treasured objects, and anything else they can get their hands on. Some children also bite, kick, hit, and scratch as they let loose full force in releasing their often intense feelings.

Difficulty paying attention and following directions   These children seem to live in another world. Anything can distract them from the task at hand: petting the dog, flipping on the TV, bothering a sibling, picking up a favorite toy, or eating a gumdrop. Every moment is full of endless opportunities for diversion. Just putting on socks can be an all-morning affair, not to mention something really complicated like eating breakfast.

Complaints from preschool teachers   This is often the time when teachers and caregivers begin to report problems with acting silly; inability to stop talking, follow directions, or take naps; talking back to the teacher; and getting into fights with other kids. Teachers may complain that these kids are either switched completely on (full speed ahead) or completely off (zoned out).

Mean to animals and other children   Hamsters, dogs, cats, and other small animals flee in terror from some of these youngsters, who have no idea why Muffy will not come near them anymore. We have heard of several unfortunate hamsters that have met their ends at the hands of an overzealous petite caretaker who did not understand the law of gravity. Brothers, sisters, and small friends fare little better, getting hit by a flailing fist or foot or tripped, often just for being in the proximity of their rambunctious and oblivious playmate.

Mischievous   ADHD children can be instigators and clowns, teasing and mischievous. Their silliness is contagious. They poke, hide, play tricks, climb on the teacher's desk, crawl under the tables, steal food, and make a nuisance of themselves, generally to attract attention, even if it is unfavorable.

Significant Problems Start at School

When your child is five to twelve years old and starts to attend school, many symptoms of ADHD become even more obvious, especially in the classroom. The child is likely to find a school environment more rigid and demanding than what he or she has previously faced. Problems are also more likely to surface at home as your child has to cope with more responsibilities, such as household chores and homework.

Difficulty with reading, writing, and taking tests— poor grades   Adequate reading ability and comprehension and legible handwriting may seem beyond the reach of an ADHD child. Because she has difficulties with attention and memory, she may find it hard to write and also to express herself. Distraction, impulsivity, and restlessness are not useful qualities at test time. Even if a child starts out getting good grades, the grades often drop lower and lower with time, as the material becomes more complex.

Problems following directions and completing assignments   Distractibility, daydreaming, and inability to finish what they start cause particular problems when those problems are compounded with losing interest quickly and being drawn to activities that look more immediately gratifying. These children may lose track of the original task completely.

Forgetting to turn in homework—losing things   Even if a child is able to finish his homework, he may find turning it into the teacher to be an ordeal. These kids also have a tendency to misplace other important items, such as clothes, keys, books, report cards, lunch, and money, either temporarily or irretrievably.

Spacing out   "Earth to Kevin" is often heard as parents attempt to make contact with their child, who is off exploring his or her own private galaxy of internal stimuli. Dreaminess and inattention cause the ADHD child to miss important information, social interactions, and even danger signals in the environment. These are hallmarks of ADHD children, with or without hyperactivity.

Annoying, repetitive, or clowning behavior   Fiddling and fidgeting, repetitive movements, questioning, or tapping are usually out of the conscious control of an ADHD child. Such habits, as well as intentional attention-seeking behavior, are usually off-putting to other children and adults alike, the result being reprimands or criticism.

Interrupting and blurting out   Children with ADHD often have the annoying habit of breaking into any conversation at any time. This leads children to get in trouble for inappropriate interruptions, both at home and at school.

Missing social cues, lack of friends, isolation   A big problem for ADHD kids is lack of friends. They may be slower to catch on in social situations and are often considered obnoxious, annoying, or overwhelming. Other children make fun of them, exclude them from groups and games, and rarely invite them to parties or overnights. As a result, the ADHD child experiences isolation and feelings of rejection that can last an entire lifetime or at least until it is understood and overcome by years of psychotherapy.

Physically awkward and clumsy   Being chosen for sports and games and being good in physical education classes is dependent on focused attention and physical coordination, skills that ADHD children often lack. They make up in energy what they lack in coordination, but can give up in frustration and despair.

Complaints from teachers   Parents frequently receive a constant stream of reports or calls from school about their children with ADHD. These kids can cause many problems for teachers who are trying to maintain a focused classroom environment. They need closer supervision and demand much more attention than the average child. Teachers typically complain that such children are disruptive, inattentive, difficult to discipline, and not living up to their potential.

Defiance Nearly half of the children with ADHD exhibit oppositional, defiant behavior. This can range from mildly mischievous testing to persistent, insolent, and even violent refusal to obey. This type of behavior is generally quick to pose problems at school as well as at home. It may be accompanied by lying, stealing, and striking out physically.

Aggravating Adolescents

ADHD during the teen years often has its greatest impact on school performance. This is a time of preparing for college or work life independent of the family, dating, starting to drive, and being exposed to peer pressure regarding drugs, alcohol, and sex. Although these challenges face any adolescent, they are often more daunting for those with ADHD due to the chronic faulty judgment, impulsiveness, exaggerated need for attention, and social immaturity.

Poor grades, failed tests and classes, disinterest in school—truancy Failure in school leads to disinterest and avoidance, skipping school, and eventual expulsion or quitting school before graduation. Many adolescents are tired of school and think they are ready for independent life, but the ADHD adolescent who has not learned very much in school is particularly unprepared for the challenges awaiting him.

Depression because of poor self-image   It is hard to maintain a positive self-image when confused, failing in school, and not making it socially at a time when success and image can be so vitally important. Teenagers can be prone to withdrawing and withholding their innermost feelings and self-doubts from their parents, a practice that can mask even serious depression.

Increased defiance, anger, and rebelliousness   Lack of success with school and peers can make parents or teachers lay down the law, provoking a response of anger, defiance, and acting out in opposition to authority. Impulsive acts of rebellion make the adolescent with ADHD feel as if he has some control over his own life, when he is actually failing to cope with increasingly challenging demands for performance and self-control.

Destructive behaviors   Frustration and anger can lead these youth to lash out against objects and people. Destructiveness, automobile accidents, and abusive or violent behavior toward friends and family can trigger serious repercussions.

Drug and alcohol abuse   Adolescents may abuse drugs or alcohol in a misguided attempt to numb their pain and loosen up. Alcohol, hallucinogens, opiates, barbiturates, and even amphetamines, such as Ritalin itself, may be used for stimulation or to reduce the pain of adolescent struggles, in some cases leading to lifelong addictions.

Difficulties or failure in jobs   Inability to focus, carry out tasks effectively, follow directions, and think clearly can lead to failure in jobs at just the time when positive reinforcement and success is crucially important. At this point, it becomes evident just how limiting and damaging a teen's ADHD can be.

Need for constant stimulation   Bored easily, the ADHD adolescent seeks constant stimulation and adventure, whether in the form of loud music, fast cars, shoplifting, or abuse of drugs and alcohol. Restlessness and impulsivity take less the form of fidgeting and more the form of adventure-seeking and risk-taking activities

Isolation and limited social skills   The social problems of ADHD are compounded by peer pressure and awakening sexuality. Where social cues are often subtle, and it is so easy to feel teased and excluded, the ADHD teenager often finds herself on the outside of her social circle looking in, without friends or dates. These adolescents may find themselves at a loss to know what to do to fit in and be accepted.

Special Challenges for Adults with ADHD

Tough times with work and career   The pressures of deadlines, tardiness, failure to complete work assignments, spacing out on the job, talking without thinking, making impulsive decisions, or acting inappropriately in the workplace can create a pattern of repetitive failure and eventual dismissal. The job history of individuals with ADHD often shows a succession of jobs lasting a short time.

Low self-esteem   The net effect of years of inattention, compromised achievement, and hyperactivity with the resulting feelings of failure, criticism, and disapproval can be devastating. Being unable to measure up academically can be damaging to one's aspirations, morale, and career potential.

Limited social skills   Socially immature and tending to behave inappropriately, many adults with ADHD find themselves unable to establish and maintain satisfying relationships, no matter how hard they try. The result is frustration, depression, anxiety, and low self-esteem for these people, even though they may be highly intelligent and well intentioned.

Difficulty with reading, learning, concentration, and memory   As the demands of adult life increase, the ability to read, write, focus, learn, and master new tasks is increasingly challenging for ADHD adults. Their academic deficits catch up with them as they find themselves performing mental tasks less skillfully than the other adults with whom they are competing in the marketplace.

Losing things—forgetting to complete daily tasks
Adults continue to lose and forget possessions and tasks, leading to disappointment with themselves and disapproval from others. Regularly, they may forget keys, checkbooks, important mail, credit cards, and appointments.

Absentmindedness and daydreaming   Earth is still trying to contact Kevin years or decades later. Adults with ADHD may continue to be drifty, dreamy, and spacey and may find the workaday, humdrum nature of routine life to be an annoying intrusion upon their fantasies.

Seek out constant stimulation, change, and immediate gratification   Changing jobs, changing relationships, or homes can be fruitless attempts to combat boredom with distraction and greener pastures. As part of the ongoing boredom syndrome, these folks may expect immediate satisfaction or they will move on to something else.

Unfulfilled potential   ADHD adults may be hard-pressed to communicate effectively, to know and choose what they really want to do with their lives, and to channel their talents into effective avenues of expression. Unable to either identify or carry out their desires, they become frustrated and despondent.

3

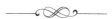

Epidemic or Overdiagnosis?
Can So Many Children
Have ADHD?

Few diagnoses are as controversial as ADHD. Some psychiatrists and psychologists, including Thomas Armstrong, Ph.D., author of *The Myth of the ADHD Child,* consider the very concept of ADHD a means of social control aimed at forcing children to behave in a particular, narrowly defined manner.[2] Peter Breggin, M.D., author of *Talking Back to Ritalin* and *Toxic Psychiatry,*[3] holds a similar view. Dr. Breggin, a radical psychiatrist, refuses even to acknowledge the diagnosis of ADHD, much less prescribe Ritalin.[4]

A second group of professionals acknowledges that many children do indeed have symptoms that correspond to the diagnosis of ADHD. They contend, how-

---

[2] Thomas Armstrong, Ph.D., *The Myth of the ADD Child* (New York: Dutton, 1995).

[3] Peter R. Breggin, M.D., *Talking Back to Ritalin: What Doctors Aren't Telling You About Stimulants for Children* (Common Courage Press, 1998) and *Toxic Psychiatry* (New York: St. Martin's, 1994).

[4] The Merrow Report: *ADD—A Dubious Diagnosis.* Public Broadcasting System. October 20, 1994.

ever, that the condition is either overdiagnosed or is an adaptive response to an overstimulated society. Dr. Stanley Greenspan, author of *The Challenging Child,* insists that some attention problems due to visual, auditory, motor, and spacial processing difficulties are often misdiagnosed as ADHD.[5] In *Attention Deficit Disorder: A Different Perception* and *ADD Success Stories,* Thom Hartmann prefers to look at ADHD as a creative, adaptive response by the descendants of hunters compelled to live in a farmers' world.[6] Richard DeGrandpre, in *Ritalin Nation: Rapid-Fire Culture* and *The Transformation of Human Consciousness,* makes a compelling argument for ADHD as the consequence of living in a stimuli-saturated culture.[7]

We agree more with this second group. We acknowledge that many children do manifest symptoms included in the diagnostic entity of ADHD, that some of these children are inadequately diagnosed, and that the growing number of children classified with ADHD is alarming. We have definitely seen cases of children in rigid classrooms or family situations, where social control does come into play. At the same time, however, we have treated many other children in more relaxed learning and home environments who also have ADHD. We have seen far too many excessively rambunctious youngsters in our office who literally cannot sit still or

---

[5] Stanley Greenspan, Ph.D., *The Challenging Child* (Reading, MA: Addison-Wesley, 1995).

[6] Thom Hartmann, *Attention Deficit Disorder: A Different Perception* (Grass Valley, CA: Underwood Books, 1995) and *ADD Success Stories* (Grass Valley, CA: Underwood Books, 1995).

[7] Richard DeGrandpre, *Ritalin Nation: Rapid-Fire Culture* (New York: W.W. Norton, 1999) and *The Transformation of Human Consciousness* (New York: W.W. Norton, 1999).

keep their hands off everything in sight to discount the diagnosis entirely. Yet we have also met many a child diagnosed with ADHD who, in our opinion, really has other problems such as learning disabilities or anxiety, or for whom ADHD is actually more of a secondary than a primary problem.

A Spoonful of Serotonin??

Most psychiatrists, psychologists, and mental-health professionals attribute ADHD, depression, obsessive-compulsive disorder, and most other mental and emotional problems to an imbalance in neurotransmitters within the brain, often serotonin or dopamine. These substances allow nerves to transmit information chemically from once cell to another. Many studies have attempted to correlate ADHD with specific neurotransmitter abnormalities. A group of researchers from the University of Georgia reviewed these neuroanatomical, neurochemical, and neurophysiological theories and studies.[8] They concluded that although the evidence does suggest neurological differences in children diagnosed with ADHD, their significance and precise mechanism remains unknown. The authors recommended a differential diagnosis of ADHD, learning disability, and conduct disorder. They suggest that it may be more accurate to view the syndrome as a cluster of various behavioral deficits, including attention, hyperactivity, and impulsivity, which share a common response to psychostimulants.

Even if a specific neurotransmitter *were* definitively associated with ADHD, we, as homeopaths, would still

---

[8] C.A. Ricco *et al.,* "Neurological Basis of Attention Deficit Hyperactivity Disorder." *Exceptional Children* 60: 118–124 (1993).

not consider this imbalance the underlying problem. Whether the disease is ADHD, a sore throat traced to streptococcus, or asthma, we identify the underlying problem as the vulnerability of each individual due to a *fundamental* lack of balance on the energetic level. Once a person is brought into equilibrium, *all* of these symptoms will improve without having to resort to a different drug for each problem.

Like Parent, Like Child

We see many children who are the spitting image of their parents. The mothers or fathers may also have had difficulty with reading or concentration, although most often they were not formally diagnosed with attention or learning problems. Boys may demonstrate the same explosive tempers and total lack of patience as their angry fathers. Some of the most worn-out parents we have encountered are those who have two, three, or even more kids bouncing off the walls. We remember one child whose chief problem was absentmindedness, despite his brilliant intellect. He devoured books about atoms and quarks, and his favorite pastime was contemplating the boundlessness of the universe. His father was the same way: a remarkable visionary who could scarcely remember to change his socks. His paternal grandfather, a nationally renowned physicist, had suffered repeated car accidents because he couldn't be bothered to keep his car on the road.

Many experts have documented a genetic contribution to ADHD, ranging from 50 to 80 percent, depending on the study or opinion.[9] Researchers at the University

[9] Lawrence Diller, *Running on Ritalin: A Physician Reflects on Children, Society, and Performance in a Pill* (New York: Bantam, 1998).

of California, Irvine reported finding the first abnormal gene associated with ADHD. The gene controls dopamine receptors in the brain. Children with a more severe form of ADHD have an abnormality of this gene, causing less sensitivity to dopamine, a neurotransmitter. Ritalin is known to stimulate dopamine release, perhaps accounting for the drug's efficacy.[10]

However, there is no radiologic, biochemical, neurophysiological, or neuropsychological test for ADHD to compare the prevalence in parent and child.[11] As a result, we still have no way of knowing just what ADHD traits are passed on through the genes and which are mimicked or learned by years of example. Not all kids, however, are holographic images of their parents. In some cases, wild, tantrumming, climbing-the-wall children have the mellowest parents. They exhibit these extreme behaviors despite living in a safe and loving environment, and the parents have made conscientious efforts to limit exposure to television, guns, violent movies, computer games, and sugar. Go figure!

ADHD: Acute Digital, High-Tech Delirium

There is no doubt in our minds that the insanely rapid pace of our sound-byte-a-minute society has contributed to the dramatic increase in the number of children diag-

---

[10] "Study Links Gene Abnormality to Hyperactive Children," *Seattle Times,* May 1, 1996.

[11] Larry Goldman, Myron Genel, Rebecca Bezman, and Priscilla Slanetz, "Diagnosis and Treatment of Attention-Deficit/Hyperactivity Disorder in Children and Adults." *Journal of the American Medical Association* 279(14): 1106 (1998).

nosed with ADHD. We live in the most overstimulated society on the planet. Most kids these days would much rather zoom home from school to absorb their minds in Nintendo rather than run track or swim laps, both of which would serve much better to release their pent-up energy. Many children are glued to the television set. Movies, even previews, are speedy, scary, and filled with ever more technologically advanced depictions of gratuitous and graphic violence. We eat fast, play fast, and can never seem to get anywhere fast enough. Our social interactions often take place in fast-food restaurants that are decorated in jangly colors that encourage customers to wolf down food hurriedly and move on in order to make space for the next relay team. We down caffeine, double espressos, and prescription and street drugs to keep up the impossible pace. Even those of us who have sworn off coffee may use highly stimulating herbs, including ma huang and guarana, that contain ephedra or up to seven times as much caffeine as coffee. Our society places precious little value on tranquility, silence, solitude, and the simple joy of being in nature.

Is ADHD a Dietary Problem?

Parents often tell us that their child's behavior is considerably worse the morning after Halloween or any other sugar binge. The perceptions of these parents have recently been supported by researchers at the Yale University School of Medicine. They found that within a few hours after substantial sugar intake, children release large amounts of adrenaline, which causes them to experience shakiness, anxiety, excitement, and concentration problems. Their brain waves also indicated a decreased ability to focus.[12] As naturopathic physicians with considerable training in nutrition, we are appalled that, per capita, Americans consume more than 130 pounds of sugar per year. Worse yet, children are notorious fast-food, carbohydrate-overloaded junkies. We are aware that some parents attribute their children's behavioral and learning problems to food and environmental allergies, salicylates, artificial colors, flavorings, additives, and preservatives. Yet a review of the literature indicated that the Feingold diet—which severely restricts these substances—has helped only a small percentage of children with ADHD.[13] Undoubtedly, for some children, allergy elimination diet or strict Feingold diet (which eliminates all salicylates as well as artificial colors and additives) is quite effective. Their parents have no need to seek out homeopathy. We believe that, although dietary factors can *exacerbate* an already existing tendency to certain behavioral or learning problems, they are not the *cause*.

For multiple reasons, we prefer to rely on homeopathy rather than on dietary changes as our primary approach to treating ADHD. We certainly encourage a healthy diet that emphasizes whole, natural foods. Nevertheless, we have seen many children with attention, behavior, and learning problems who, despite eliminating cow's milk, wheat, and other foods from their diets, have *not* experienced a consistent and significant improvement. Second, parents of ADHD kids can become burned out just riding herd on them to brush their teeth

---

[12] *Journal of Pediatrics*, February, 1996 cited in *Well Being Journal*, May/June 1996.

[13] E.H. Wender, "The Food Additive-Free Diet in the Treatment of Behavior Disorders: A Review," *Developmental and Behavioral Pediatrics* 7: 35–42 (1986).

or get dressed for school; they might well be over-whelmed if the also attempted to radically restrict their diets. Third, many of these children already feel stigma-tized because of their social awkwardness, learning dif-ficulties, and disruptive behaviors. If they are required to eat different foods than all the other children, they may feel even more strange and different. Fourth, since homeopathy treats the whole child, sensitivities to foods or environmental factors are likely to be much less of a problem after the child has been brought into balance through homeopathy. Lastly, the degree of transforma-tion in attention, behavior, social skills, grades, physical health, and overall happiness that we have witnessed with homeopathy are much greater than what we be-lieve to be possible through dietary change alone.

What About the Social Control Issue?

How valid are criticisms that the overdiagnosis of ADHD is a means for teachers to control unruly, high-spirited children who tend to disrupt a well-run class-room? Four years and nearly two thousand patients since we wrote the first edition of *Ritalin-Free Kids,* we wish we had more favorable comments on the subject of teachers overstepping their bounds. When we first heard the reports of parents threatened with their chil-dren's expulsion from a particular classroom unless they were put on Ritalin, we could hardly believe our ears. How, we wondered, was this legal? It must be the rare teacher who would exert so much pressure on al-ready stressed-out parents of ADHD kids. But we have heard this same story again and again. In the most ex-treme cases, parents are invited for a conference with the teacher, only to find themselves in a room crowded with the principal, psychologist, special-education teacher, occupational therapist, and, of course, the teacher. In such scenarios, all of the invited professional guests echo the same refrain: "Your child is unmanageable and needs Ritalin."

We do sympathize with the teachers who are generally overworked, underpaid, and charged with the overwhelming, often thankless, task of educating challenging children in overflowing classrooms. Thinking of ways to deal with one or more disruptive, learning-disabled, defiant, overstimulated children in a classroom of thirty is no piece of cake. However, we do not agree that the answer lies in pressuring the parents of these children to subject their children to medication when the parent is not in agreement. There are many other alternatives, such as IEPs (individual education plans), tutoring, family therapy, and nondrug interventions, including homeopathy or neurofeedback. Teachers are not doctors and should not be in the role of diagnosing ADHD, much less suggesting stimulant medication. ADHD is a multifactorial problem that requires parents, educators, health care providers, and, above all, the children themselves to work together.

Gifted or Hyperactive?

Some people are surprised to learn that precocious children may be included in the ADHD category and have been known to end up in a special-education classroom designed for kids with learning problems. Ask yourself, if you had an IQ of 150 and a photographic memory, how well would you tolerate a regular fourth-grade classroom? You would probably be bored to tears unless your teacher created special activities and outlets for your unusual intellectual capabilities. You might tap your pencil on your desk, design paper skyscrapers, or invent a magical world of dinosaurs.

James Webb and Diane Latimer address this dilemma: "In the classroom, a gifted child's perceived inability to stay on task might be related to boredom, curriculum, mismatched learning style, or other environmental factors. Gifted children may spend from one-fourth to one-half of their regular classroom time waiting for others to catch up—even more if they are in a heterogeneously grouped class."[14] Because a gifted child may demonstrate ADHD-like behaviors in some settings and not others, one classroom teacher may label her with ADHD while the other teachers do not. The authors recommend individual evaluation followed by appropriate curricular and instructional changes to account for advanced knowledge, diverse learning styles, and various types of intelligence. Such individual evaluation is exactly what homeopathy has to offer.

A Matter of Predisposition

Other than saying that anyone with ADHD must have a predisposition to it, be it hereditary or environmental, it is fruitless to ascribe all of the individual ADHDs to one cause. Each of us, with or without ADHD, is one of a kind. Even if a child has two parents with ADHD and plays video games and devours sugar all day, he may or may not ever develop ADHD. How is this possible? Homeopaths believe that the reason some children and

---

[14] James T. Webb and Diane Latimer, "ADHD and Children Who Are Gifted," *ERIC Digest*, #E522 (1993).

adults suffer from ADHD and others do not lies in susceptibility or predisposition. If you ask the mother of a child with ADHD when she first noticed problem behaviors or tendencies in her child, she will likely say infancy or toddlerhood. Such a child may have been hyperalert and tended to wake frequently during the night, to be fussy and hard to satisfy, to run as soon as he could walk, and to climb all over the furniture as soon as he was mobile. This predisposition to ADHD-like behavior often occurs at a very tender age. Homeopaths frequently observe that this tendency depends on the constitution of the individual from birth and may even be affected by the state of the parents prior to conception and during pregnancy.

Most important to a homeopath are the unique tendencies or predispositions of the individual child or adult, regardless of what specifically may trigger the susceptibility. The phenomenon of susceptibility varies from individual to individual and cannot be stereotyped. But a homeopath listens carefully to everything the person communicates and attempts to understand her thoroughly. From this process, a homeopathic medicine is selected, which should shift that susceptibility and bring about balance and healing.

4

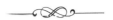

The ADHD Pressure Cooker
Kids, Teachers, Parents, and Doctors
All Feel the Heat

Put Yourself in Any of Their Shoes

What has impressed us the most in treating large numbers of children with behavioral and learning problems, the majority of them diagnosed with ADHD, is their intensity. We are equally struck by how easily that intensity, tension, and pressure is passed on from one member of the ADHD child's network to the next, including us. Parents most frequently use the word "desperate." It is a sense of urgency, a fix-this-child-fast mentality that parents, teachers, and caregivers often share. Even though ADHD by itself is not life threatening and is truly physically dangerous only in the case of accompanying conditions such as serious drug addiction, homicidal anger, or suicidal impulses, a sense of urgency and immediacy nevertheless permeates the condition.

The behaviors associated with ADHD, particularly in its moderate to severe forms, are not easy for anyone to live with, least of all the child or adult suffering from it. The child, who in some way is not happy or comfortable in his own skin, sets off a type of chain reaction. He can't control his impulses, words, or actions and consequently irritates, disturbs, aggravates, or infuriates those around him, depending on which of *their* buttons is pushed. It might be a teacher who is already trying to manage thirty other little rug rats or testy teenagers, a parent who is overworked, underpaid, and underappreciated, a babysitter who fights her own impulse to smack her little charges, or a physician who is pushed to prescribe medications that she may or may not believe are indicated for that child.

The bottom line: It's not easy for children who have been diagnosed with ADHD. They know how frustrated they make everyone around them, but they just can't figure out a way to be "normal" and acceptable. The teachers feel like screaming and may react punitively out of their own performance stress and anxiety. The parents simply want some peace and quiet and to do what is best for their child. The caregivers want to do their best for the child to the extent their patience allows. The doctors may feel compelled to prescribe medications without sufficient information or conviction. Welcome to the ADHD pressure cooker!

Nick: The child with ADHD   My name is Nick, and I am an eight-year-old in the second grade. I'm kind of nervous about doing my homework right, doing okay on tests, and getting good reports from my teacher. I want to please my parents so they'll be proud of me and will let me watch my favorite TV shows, play video games whenever I want, and have my friends over for sleepovers or to play.

But my parents don't seem very happy with me. They're constantly telling me to do the same thing a million times over, then yelling at me when I forget it again. They tell me that I'm zoning out, not listening to them, not doing what they tell me to do. I try, but it just doesn't seem to make a difference. I don't *want* to make them mad, but whatever they tell me to do just flies out of my mind. And they tell me too many things at the same time. How can anybody remember to do five different things at the same time? I didn't mean to leave my brand new jacket at school where it never turned up again, or to forget to bring home my notebook with all my assignments in it, or to spill grape juice on my mom's new champagne-colored sofa. These things just *happen* to me.

Then there's my older sister, Sasha, and my little brother, Sky. I don't *mean* to bug them and get on their nerves. I don't *try* to tap my feet and move around all the time and ask too many questions. Or to break their favorite toys or go into their rooms when they don't want me there. It's not my fault that my mom and dad have to spend so much extra time trying to help me with my homework that there's not much time left for them. Why do they seem so mad at me, and why does Sasha make me feel like she wishes I weren't even around?

It's not much better in the friends department. Nobody likes me and I never get invited to birthday parties like the other kids. I eat lunch by myself and there's nobody to play with at recess. They just make fun of me and don't pick me for their teams.

And then there's school. I really don't think Mrs. Claremont likes me either. Whenever she calls on me, my mind is off somewhere else and I don't know the answer. Or I get in trouble for clicking my pencil or tapping my feet when I'm just bored. It seems like Mrs. Claremont is always mad at me for something I'm doing or not doing. I didn't *mean* to lose those homework assignments or to not be able to finish my tests. And she never has anything nice to say on the notes she sends home. They usually get me grounded or I lose my allowance for the whole week.

I guess I don't like myself any more than anybody else likes me. No matter how hard I try, I still feel like a loser.

Mrs. Claremont: Second-grade teacher   This is my eleventh year of teaching, and this is the toughest class yet! Not only did they give me a class of thirty kids, but they also cut my aides down to one, and she's brand new and not much help. They expect me to do a great teaching job, and I want to help those kids. That's why I went into teaching in the first place. But it seems to get harder and harder every year!

It used to be that I had one difficult kid in my class, and now I have four. Two have IEPs and get taken out of class at various times, and at least two others need IEPs. The kids are so much harder to control than they used to be. Either they won't stay in their seats or they don't care about learning or they're moving around incessantly. Those three kids with ADHD are so distractible that they keep the other kids from learning. I don't know how to make them sit still. When I went into teaching, nobody told me I'd have to be a policewoman to make sure they don't bring guns to school or that I'd have to spend have my time just telling them to stay in their seats and keep their mouths shut.

I really don't know what to do with Nick. He's a nice kid, but he drives me crazy. Can't sit quietly at his desk to save his life and blurts out the answers before anyone else has a chance to say anything. That kid can't remember to take home his assignment sheets, much less turn in his homework. I don't see how he'll pass second grade unless he shapes up. I just don't have time to give him the kind of attention that he needs. It's been a month since the school year started, and he still isn't catching on. I think he has ADHD. His parents need to put him on Ritalin. And if they don't want to, and he keeps up like this, I just can't have him in my class.

Betty and Jim: Nick's parents   We love Nick and want him to do the very best he can. We know he's a good kid, but we worry about him. He's absent-minded, loses everything in sight, and is weak on follow-through. We just can't figure out why he can't concentrate. We never had this problem when we were in school. All that seems to hold Nick's attention is Nintendo and Pokémon. And the other kids give him such a hard time. His self-esteem is down the tubes.

We've read about ADHD, and it does seem to fit him, but the idea of giving him amphetamines isn't very appealing. He's already thin, and we're afraid he'll lose even more weight. And it's already hard for him to get a good night's sleep. But what should we do? Are we being unfair to him if we don't give him stimulants? Depriving him of his ability to succeed?

You read so much about ADHD these days. How overdiagnosed it is and how they're giving kids all kinds of medications that have only been tested on adults. And the huge jump in Ritalin production, most of which is used in the U.S. We know the school will start pushing us to have Nick diagnosed with ADHD and get stimulants. That's what we hear from the parents of other kids like Nick. But what if he ever wants to go in the military? He won't be accepted later if we give him Ritalin now. What do we do?

Bill Murphy: Nick's pediatrician So, here's Nick. A nice kid with a case of moderate ADHD. His parents aren't pressuring me to prescribe Ritalin, like often happens in my practice. He hasn't had a psychological workup, but he certainly does have the symptoms. Funny how many kids seem to have ADHD these days. It wasn't like that when I started out fifteen years ago. Kids seemed much more normal back then. Ear infections, strep throats—I hardly ever saw a case of ADHD. And now millions of kids out there are on Ritalin. And more on Prozac or Clonodine.

I want to do the best for Nick, but what does that mean? Give him Ritalin till he outgrows the ADHD, if he ever does? Refuse and let his parents find another doctor who will? Make some other suggestion? Ritalin is very likely to help him. I haven't read about anything else that seems as effective.

An Epidemic of ADHD?

Every member of this scenario is under pressure and has his or her own needs. This situation is far too common. Indeed, it is so common that a recent study in *Pediatrics* found that nearly three times as many children in the United States have emotional or behavioral problems as did twenty years ago.[15] Since 1990 the number of children and adults in the United States diagnosed with ADHD has increased from under one million to five million. The amount of Ritalin produced in the United States during the same time frame has risen 700 per-

---

[15] Reuters and the Associated Press, "Doctors See Big Increase in Troubled Children: Study Cites Stressed-Out Families," *The Seattle Times,* June 6, 2000, A1.

cent.[16] Ritalin, or methylphenidate, is an amphetamine created in 1955 that now accounts for 90 percent of the stimulant use in ADHD in this country.[17] Hundreds of studies have documented the short-term benefits of stimulant medications in the treatment of ADHD, but evidence remains lacking that demonstrates their long-term benefits on school achievement, peer relations, or behavior problems in adolescents.[18] Accusations of over-diagnosis and overmedication of preschoolers for ADHD has prompted the federal government to fund a $5 million research project to study children who are taking Ritalin.[19] For the same reason, the Colorado Board of Education passed a resolution urging teachers to rely on discipline and instruction to handle behavior problems in the classroom and discouraging them recommending medical evaluations for ADHD and treatment with Ritalin.[20]

Ritalin Is Not the Only Answer

The problem here is that few people faced with the problem are aware of other possibilities. It's Ritalin (or another pharmaceutical drug) or nothing. This outlook

[16] Lawrence Diller, *Running on Ritalin: A Physician Reflects on Children, Society, and Performance in a Pill* (New York: Bantam, 1998), 2.

[17] Goldman *et al.*, op. cit., 1103.

[18] D. Jacobvitz *et al.*, as cited in G. LeFever *et al.*, "The Extent of Drug Therapy for Attention Deficit-Hyperactivity Disorder Among Children in Public Schools." *American Journal of Public Health* 89(9): 1363 (1999).

[19] N. Anderson, "U.S. Pledges Hard Look at Use of Behavior Drugs on Children," *The Seattle Times,* March 21, 2000, A4.

[20] M. Janofsky, "Behavior Drugs for the Young Debated Anew," *New York Times,* November 25, 1999, 1.

is encouraged by Novartis, the manufacturer of Ritalin, and CHADD (Children and Adults with ADD), the nationwide support group that provides most of the education for parents of kids with ADHD. The majority of child and behavioral psychiatrists and psychologists and some pediatricians also support Ritalin use. Few, even those who believe that ADHD is overdiagnosed and Ritalin overprescribed, will consider the possibility that non-drug alternatives outside of behavioral therapy or, possibly, neurofeedback, may be effective.

We urge those who are looking for a safe, effective, and natural answer to ADHD and other behavioral and learning problems, to at least consider the possibility that homeopathy may work for you or your child.

Children and adults with ADHD, teachers, parents, and physicians are all under duress to find quick answers for this not-so-straightforward problem. They all deserve information, support, and time to make the best decisions possible. We encourage them to do so with an open mind.

5

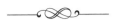

To Drug or Not to Drug
The Pros and Cons of Conventional Treatment for ADHD and Other Behavioral and Mood Disorders

Over Ten Million Stimulant Prescriptions for Kids

Picture a line of energetic, rambunctious kids lining up at noon at school. Is it lunchtime? Yes. Are these children waiting their turn in the cafeteria queue? No, they are lining up for drugs doled out by a secretary or, in the wealthier school districts, a school nurse. Ritalin is short acting, wearing off after four hours or so. Overamped kids often take one dose in the morning, a second at lunchtime, and a third when they return from school, depending on the child's behavior, the action of the drug, and the parents' threshold. Steve Friedman, principal since 1990 of Nova Middle School in Fort Lauderdale, Florida, expressed surprise at the growing number of children in his school who were taking Ritalin. When he joined the school, the nurse handed out two prescriptions per day; by 1995 the number had risen to sixty.[21]

---

[21] The Merrow Report, op. cit.

As stated earlier, between 1990 and 1993 the number of children's outpatient visits for ADHD grew from 1.4 million to 4.2 million. Over 90 percent of those visits resulted in prescriptions. The number of office visits for children during which Ritalin (methylphenidate) was prescribed during 1995 totaled nearly two million. Total prescriptions for all stimulant drugs were nearly six million. By 1996, more than ten million prescriptions for Ritalin were written, and nearly 7 percent of American school-age children were on stimulant medication.[22] Dr. Lawrence Diller reports in his book, *Running on Ritalin,* that according to Drug Enforcement Agency (DEA) figures, Ritalin production between 1990 and 1997 in the United States increased more than 700 percent.[23] These figures and similar statistics have become cause for alarm that too many children are being given these potent medications for ADHD and related disorders.

Off-Label Drugs for Toddlers

The problem of overprescription of psychotropic medications is not limited to Ritalin or other stimulants used to treat ADHD. Children are being given a number of psychiatric prescriptions that are considered off-label, meaning that the medications have not been tested on or approved by the Food and Drug Administration (FDA) for use by children. Physicians are prescribing these drugs for conditions that often occur with ADHD,

---

[22] Laurence Greenhill, Jeffrey Halperin, and Howard Abikoff, "Stimulant Medications," *Journal of the American Academy of Child and Adolescent Psychiatry* 38(5): 504 (1999).

[23] Lawrence Diller, op.cit., p. 34.

such as depression, Tourette's disorder, oppositional defiant disorder, conduct disorder, and anxiety disorders.

Should Prozac be given to depressed three-year-olds? To our, and surely your, amazement, this drug was actually given to 3,000 children under one year old in 1995.[24] When does a child's opposition cease to be normal behavior and become a disorder? When should normal levels of activity for preschoolers be termed hyperactive? These questions, and other issues relating to overdiagnosis and overprescription of medication, led First Lady Hillary Clinton in the spring of 2000 to call for more research on pediatric dosing and Ritalin use in preschoolers. She also urged the National Institutes of Mental Health and the Department of Education to provide more facts to parents who must decide whether to medicate their children.

The types of medications being given to children are astounding. Stimulants, antihypertensive drugs, tricyclic and SSRI antidepressants, antianxiety agents, antiepileptics, mood stabilizers, and antipsychotic drugs, singly or in combination. Many of these drugs have never been approved for use in children. Although not illegal, this off-label use is controversial. According to a February 2000 article in the *Journal of the American Medical Association,* "Controlled clinical studies to evaluate the efficacy of psychotropic medications for preschoolers are rare. Efficacy data are essentially lacking for clonidine and the SSRIs and methylphenidate's adverse effects for preschool children are more pronounced than for older youths. Consequently, the vast

---

[24] Julio Zito, Daniel Safer, Susan dosReis, James Gardner, Myde Boles, and Frances Lynch, "Trends in the Prescribing of Psychotropic Medications to Preschoolers." *Journal of the American Medical Association* 283(8): 1025–1030 (2000).

majority of psychotropic medications prescribed for preschoolers are being used off-label."[25] That same week, *Newsweek* reported that Dr. Steve Hyman, director of the National Institute of Mental Health, was shocked that physicians increasingly appear to be using clonidine, a drug used to treat high blood pressure in adults, to treat ADHD symptoms or insomnia. He also expressed great concern that the physicians are prescribing the older generation of tricyclic antidepressants for preschoolers. Clonidine in combination with stimulants has been associated with heart problems in children. And there's no evidence that tricyclics, which can also have serious side effects, even work for depression in kids. Tricyclics are also used to control impulses and treat bedwetting. "But in children so young," says Hyman. "I don't see a justification for using them."[26]

To Speed or Not to Speed

Although a comprehensive treatment plan for ADHD may include behavior modification, cognitive therapy, family therapy, and training in social skills, stimulant medication is the mainstay of conventional treatment of ADHD. The principal drugs used are as Ritalin (methylphenidate), Dexedrine (dextroamphetamine), or the mixed amphetamine preparation, Adderall. Other stimulants such as Desoxyn and Cylert (pemoline) are rarely used due to their side effects. Cylert, for example, has been known to cause liver damage. Ritalin, Dexedrine, and Adderall are all Schedule II controlled substances,

[25] Zito *et al.,* op. cit., p. 1028.

[26] Claudia Kalb, "Drugged-Out Toddlers," *Newsweek,* March 6, 2000, 53.

requiring special prescribing practices and careful control.[27] These drugs affect neurotransmitter release in the brain, allowing better use of dopamine and norepinephrine in those centers involved in ADHD.

Ritalin is the most commonly prescribed and most researched stimulant medication for ADHD. Ritalin is an amphetamine. In both normal children and those with ADHD, it increases attention, but in ADHD children it also makes them less impulsive and hyperactive. A dose given to a child lasts about four hours, which means that many children require a midday dose for continued effectiveness or a sustained-release form for longer action. When the dose has worn off, the child may experience a rebound effect, with increased hyperactivity, restlessness, inattention, and impulsiveness. This leads many parents to also give an evening dose to control behavior. The additional medication, while helping children behave in the home, can cause other problems by increasing the chances of insomnia and appetite loss.

For children who do not respond well to Ritalin, a physician may try Dexedrine, another amphetamine that comes in a time-release form, eliminating the need for a midday dose. Dexedrine's side effects are nearly identical to those of Ritalin. Adderall, a combination of four amphetamines, has a sustained action, lasting longer than the other stimulants, up to eight hours per dose. For this reason, physicians are increasingly prescribing it for ADHD.

Children or adults with ADHD may respond to one, all, or none of the stimulant drugs. When stimulants are not effective, children may be given tricyclic or SSRI

[27] Timothy E. Wilens, *Straight Talk About Psychiatric Medications for Kids* (New York: Guilford, 1999), 195.

antidepressants, antianxiety agents, or mood stabilizers. Stimulants have a short-term effectiveness of 60 to 80 percent in reducing the hyperactivity, distractibility, and impulsiveness of school-age children.[28] Similar rates of success have been found in adults with ADHD.[29] Stimulant medications have also been shown to improve attention span, gross motor coordination, impulsivity, aggressiveness, handwriting, and compliance with requests or instructions.[30] Children have also achieved short-term learning benefits while on these medications, but no lasting improvement in academic success has been shown.

A compilation of all the review studies published during the past twenty years on the effects of stimulant medication for ADHD concluded that medication resulted in temporary management of diagnostic symptoms, including overactivity, inattention, and impulsivity, as well as increased compliance, effort, and academic productivity and decreased aggression and negative behaviors.[31] Clearly, stimulant medications work, at least in the short term. More than 200 controlled studies have been done on more than 5,000 patients.[32] Many parents and teachers heavily rely on stimulant medications to control inattentive and unruly children, at home and in the classroom. "The use of stimulant drugs results

[28] A.R. Adesman and E.H. Wender, "Helping the Hyperactive Child," *Patient Care,* March 30, 1992, 96–116.

[29] Paul H. Wender, *Attention Deficit Hyperactivity Disorder in Adults* (New York/Oxford: Oxford University Press, 1995), 166.

[30] Adesman and Wender, op. cit., 105.

[31] J.M. Swanson *et al.,* "Effect of Stimulant Medication on Children with Attention Deficit Disorder: A Review of Reviews," *Exceptional Children* 60: 154–162 (1993).

[32] Wilens, op. cit., 195.

in an immediate and often dramatic improvement in behavior. Attentiveness improves, and interpersonal interactions, including those with parents, are less confrontational. Teachers do not need to work as hard to control the children and are more approving of their behavior. Academic performance improves, but not as dramatically as behavior. Laboratory measures of attention, impulsivity, learning, information processing, short-term memory, and vigilance all improve. . . . These findings have . . . been confirmed in many controlled short-term studies . . . of children, adolescents and adults; an estimated 70 percent of the patients responded to the stimulant drugs . . . , eliminating most controversy over at least the short-term efficacy and safety of these drugs."[33]

Given the lack of consistent long-term benefits, why has stimulant medication continued to be the primary treatment for ADHD? Ritalin and other stimulants do produce significant short-term gains for a large percentage of children and adults with ADHD. These gains may be important in preserving the self-esteem of the individual with ADHD and the sanity of their teachers, families, and peers. Ritalin may have an even greater tendency to relieve stress in the caregiver than in the child.[34] The educational and social benefits of pharmaceutical behavior control are considered far greater than the risks of the medication, and conventional medicine offers no viable alternative.

[33] J. Elia, P.J. Ambrosini, and J. Rapoport, "Treatment of Attention Deficit Hyperactivity Disorder," *New England Journal of Medicine* 340:10, 783 (1999).

[34] Swanson *et al.,* op. cit., 156

Because of the well-known and documented efficacy of stimulant drugs, schoolteachers, counselors, and mental-health professionals may lean on you to medicate your child and suggest that drugs are "the right thing to do for your child." They may tell you, "If your child had an infection, you would give him antibiotics. So if he has ADHD, you need to give him stimulants." Remember, it is your own or your child's health and life that are at stake. You need to feel comfortable about the choice that you make regarding treatment.

Many children do respond positively to stimulants. However 30 percent of children with ADHD show no response to medication,[35] and a large proportion of those who respond to medication respond to a placebo as well.[36] There is no way to predict through physiological, neurological, or biochemical testing who will respond to the medication positively and who will not. The re-

The Downside of Stimulants

- Lasts only four hours to eight hours (Ritalin SR, Dexedrine spansule, or Adderall)
- Treats only some of the symptoms of ADHD
- Effective in only 70 percent of children with ADHD
- Provides only short-term superficial healing; does not treat the root of the problem
- Can cause side effects such as appetite loss, anxiety, insomnia, tics, headaches, and stomachaches
- Gets children into the habit of taking drugs
- May need to be taken throughout life

[35] Wilens, op. cit., 196.
[36] Ibid., 156

view article showed no significant improvement in reading skills, athletic or game skills, or positive social skills. Children improved less in learning and achievement than they did in behavior and attention. Overall, long-term adjustment, as measured by academic achievement, antisocial behavior, and arrest rate, was unaffected by medication.[37]

Furthermore, some people taking stimulant medication suffer from side effects. The most common are decreased appetite, weight loss, insomnia, motor tics (as in Tourette's disorder), and short-term growth retardation.[38] Some parents report other side effects, including headaches, stomachaches, increased heart rate or blood pressure, drowsiness, social withdrawal, irritability and moodiness, and involuntary movements or sounds. Stimulant medication for ADHD may be contraindicated for people with seizures, liver disease, heart disease, high blood pressure, or tic disorders. Although conventional medical opinion is that stimulants are relatively safe and effective, the possible side effects may be enough to convince you to choose another path.

Ritalin as a Street Drug

Another identified drawback of Ritalin in the last decade is its popularity as an illicit drug. The annual survey "Monitoring the Future," conducted by the University of Michigan, warns of a trend in Ritalin abuse. From 1993 to 1994 the number of high school seniors who admitted to abusing Ritalin doubled, a figure that

---

[37] Ibid., 157.

[38] R.A. Barkley and J.V. Murphy, "Treating Attention-Deficit Hyperactivity Disorder: Medication and Behavior Management Training," *Pediatric Animals* 20: 256–266 (1991).

represents about 350,000 students nationwide. Kids call Ritalin "Vitamin-R," "R-ball," or "the smart drug" and seek it out to study better and to get high.[39] A 1995 *Newsweek* article reported that students at an upscale New York college crushed and snorted Ritalin tablets like cocaine. They described an immediate rush, as if they felt hyperactive.[40]

Given this country's tremendous problem with drug addiction, the increase in abuse of Ritalin and similar drugs, which is being legally prescribed for nearly six million children, is of some concern. It is, however, less of an actual problem than it was originally expected to be, based on the trend in 1994. The manufacturers of Ritalin, in response to the reports of Ritalin abuse, sent 200,000 physicians and pharmacists pamphlets explaining the proper use of the drug.[41] Perhaps this has had the intended effect in reducing potential abuse of Ritalin and other stimulant drugs, including Dexedrine and Adderall.

Up from the Depths with Antidepressants

Physicians commonly prescribe both tricyclic and SSRI (selective serotonin reuptake inhibitors) antidepressants for children, whether or not the FDA has approved their use. "Since the release of fluoxetine (Prozac) in 1988, the use of SSRIs has been widespread. Recent reports describe more than 200,000 mentions (prescriptions, refills, etc.) of fluoxetine and sertraline (Zoloft) in 1994 for

---

[39] "Ritalin Finding Its Way Into the Schoolyard," *Seattle Times*, February 9, 1996.

[40] "A Risky Rx for Fun," *Newsweek*, October 30, 1995, 74.

[41] "Misuse of Ritalin by Schoolchildren Prompts Warning," *Seattle Times*, March 7, 1996.

children aged five to ten years. This fourfold increase in two years has led to concerns about overprescribing among children and adolescents."[42] By 1996, children six to eighteen received 735,000 prescriptions for SSRIs.[43] Obviously, the numbers are increasing dramatically. (See our book, *Prozac-Free,* for additional information on antidepressant use and alternatives.)

Tricyclic antidepressants such as amitriptyline (Elavil), desipramine (Norpramin), and imipramine (Tofranil) are not only used for childhood depression, but also to control bedwetting (nocturnal enuresis). Some children with ADHD do experience positive effects when treated with these drugs, especially those children who are not responsive to stimulants or who cannot tolerate their side effects, such as insomnia or tics.[44] Despite a good score with ADHD, the tricyclic compounds have not been proved effective for children suffering from major depressive disorders, compared with placebo, in several double-blind clinical trials. Tricyclics, however, especially clomipramine and desipramine, have been found useful in treating obsessive-compulsive disorder and ritualistic autistic behavior. Bedwetting responds quite favorably to imipramine in many, but not all cases.[45]

[42] G.J. Emslie, J.T. Walkup, S.R. Pliszka, and M. Ernst, "Non-tricyclic Antidepressants: Current Trends in Children and Adolescents." *Journal of the American Academy of Child and Adolescent Psychiatry* 38(5): 517–528 (1999).

[43] Mary Crowley, "Do Kids Need Prozac?" *Newsweek,* October 20, 1997: 73–74.

[44] Wilens, op. cit., 209.

[45] B. Geller, D. Reising, H.L. Leonard, M.A. Riddle, and B.T. Walsh, "Critical Review of Tricyclic Antidepressant Use in Children and Adolescents." *Journal of the American Academy of Child and Adolescent Psychiatry* 38(5): 513–516 (1999).

"Common short-term effects of the tricyclic anti-depressants include dry mouth, constipation, sedation, headaches, vivid dreams, stomachaches, rash and blurred vision. . . . Children on these medications also may get a red, itchy rash, usually over the chest."[46] According to Dr. Wilens, because they produce a dry mouth, the tri-cyclics also cause more tooth decay in some children. They also carry some cardiac risks, including ECG abnormalities, tachycardia, conduction problems, and the possibility in a small number of cases of sudden death of unknown origin. The greatest risk of the tricyclics is overdose, which can be lethal.

The SSRIs, a more recently developed alternative to tricyclics, have become very popular, particularly Prozac (fluoxetine), Zoloft (sertraline), Paxil (paroxetine), Celexa (Citalopram) and Luvox (fluvoxamine). All of these drugs affect the levels of serotonin, a neurotransmitter in the brain. Wellbutrin (buproprione), Effexor (venlafaxine), Serzone (nefazodone), and Desyrel (trazodone) also affect serotonin levels, but by different mechanisms. SSRIs have been found effective for the treatment of depression, anxiety, and obsessive-compulsive disorder, especially in adults, but increasingly in children. Wellbutrin has been used in cases of ADHD with a depressive component in both children and adults because it has both a stimulant and antidepressant action.

According to a review published by the American Academy of Child and Adolescent Psychiatry, the SSRIs are considered effective in children, but need more research. The authors conclude, "As in adults, also in children, nontricyclic antidepressants are potentially useful in treating a variety of psychiatric disorders. The data supporting their efficacy, however, are quite lim-

[46] Wilens, op. cit., 209–210.

ited. Obsessive-compulsive disorder is the only psychiatric diagnosis for which pediatric use of selective serotonin reuptake inhibitors has been approved. One placebo-controlled study in children and adolescents with major depression supports the efficacy of fluoxetine. Other clinical trials are in progress. One particularly disturbing side effect of Prozac on youngsters is that 6 percent of them develop mania.[47] Available data indicate that the overall safety of these medications when used by adults is good, at least in the short term. "Further research is essential to provide the necessary information on the efficacy, safety, and pharmacokinetics of these medications in children and adolescents."[48]

SSRIs may be given only once daily, which makes it more likely that people will actually take it regularly. Some are better in divided doses, twice a day. "The most common side effects of these medications include agitation, stomachaches and diarrhea, irritability, behavioral activation, headaches, insomnia and less commonly, sedation. The (SSRIs) also alter the liver's ability to break down other medications including over the counter preparations."[49] Dr. Wilens also points out that some drug interactions have been noted, particularly with Tavist (an antihistamine) and Erythromycin (an antibiotic). There are no cardiovascular side effects or need for blood level monitoring.

Heavy Drugs for Moody Kids

For ADHD children who also have unstable moods, bipolar disorder (frequently referred to as manic-depression),

[47] Crowley, op. cit., 74.

[48] Emslie *et al.*, op. cit., 517.

[49] Wilens, op. cit., 212.

or severely impulsive or aggressive behavior, physicians often prescribe mood stabilizers, including lithium carbonate and antiepileptic drugs. Lithium carbonate, Depakote (valproic acid), Neurontin, and Topamax are the most commonly used. These are potent drugs with potentially serious side effects. For extreme children, however, they can be effective and possibly worth the risk. Others would be better off with a milder alternative. (See our book, *Rage-Free Kids,* for a more thorough discussion of these children and their medications.)

In children and adolescents with bipolar disorder, as with adults, lithium is the conventional drug of choice, even though the research data is somewhat limited and researchers still do not know the mechanism of action. Common lithium side effects include nausea, diarrhea, tremor, enuresis (bedwetting), weight gain, fatigue, loss of coordination, low white cell count, and malaise. The drug can also affect the kidneys, eyes, thyroid, nervous system, skin, and cardiovascular system.[50] It is extremely important to monitor blood levels of lithium to prevent toxicity and kidney damage.

For children with very unstable moods, who may or may not be diagnosed with bipolar disorder, or for those who are more aggressive, physicians often turn to the anticonvulsants Depakote or Tegretol. These antiseizure medications have been given extensively to children, so their action and side effects are well known. They are believed to act as mood stabilizers by reducing the firing of neurons in the emotional centers of the brain.[51]

---

[50] N.D. Ryan, V.S. Bhatara, and J.M. Perel. "Mood Stabilizers in Children and Adolescents." *Journal of the American Academy of Child and Adolescent Psychiatry* 38(5): 529–536 (1999).

[51] Wilens, op. cit., 219

Tegretol use is based largely on three double-blind studies from the early 1970s. These studies indicated that Tegretol was effective in 71 of the study subjects in controlling behavioral problems or high activity levels in children. A majority of these children had abnormal EEGs. In a 1992 study, Tegretol did not help a group of twenty-two children ages five to twelve with conduct disorder who had been hospitalized for aggression. Common side effects include drowsiness, loss of coordination, and dizziness. More serious, but less common, side effects include blood disorders (aplastic anemia and agranulocytosis), and problems with the skin, liver, and pancreas. Although Tegretol has been used to treat a number of psychiatric disorders in children, the FDA has not labeled it for psychiatric use in any age group.[52]

Depakote is used for bipolar children or those with temper outbursts and moodiness. A small amount of research supports its use in adolescents, but none in children. Side effects can be significant, including sedation, nausea, dizziness and weight gain, liver toxicity, reduction in blood counts, hair loss, pancreatitis, increased blood sugar, and menstrual changes. In rare cases, children under two have suffered liver toxicity and died. In teenage women, severe metabolic and hormonal problems have been reported in one study from Finland.[53]

The effectiveness and side effects of the newer mood-stabilizing drugs—Neurontin, Lamictal, Gabitril, and Topamax—on children are not well researched yet. Thus far, however, these medications seem to have fewer and less serious side effects, the common ones being fatigue, dizziness, and unstable gait.

[52] Ryan *et al.*, op. cit., 533.
[53] Ryan *et al.*, op. cit., 535.

High-Pressure Kids on Blood Pressure Meds and Antianxiety Agents

Physicians use the antihypertensive drugs, Catapres (clonidine) and Tenex (guanfacine), extensively in the treatment of ADHD and mood and sleep problems, usually in combination with other stimulant or mood-stabilizing medications. Both Clonidine and Tenex are thought to help with hyperactivity, Tourette's and other tic disorders, and aggressiveness. No controlled studies show that clonidine is effective for ADHD. In four out of five studies of the effectiveness of clonidine, the medication had no noticeable effect. There are no controlled trials of Tenex.[54]

Tenex is considered more useful for attention problems, while clonidine is more often used for hyperactivity and aggressiveness. Side effects are minor, drowsiness being the most common. This side effect is used to advantage when a child has sleep problems or insomnia due to stimulant medications.[55]

For children with anxiety, the most common medications used are benzodiazepines such as Xanax (alprazolam) or Klonopin (clonazepam), or the newer drug, Buspar (buspirone) that works by a different mechanism. The benzodiazepines act on the GABA receptors in the central nervous system. Buspar works on influencing serotonin levels. The benzodiazepines are more effective in reducing anxiety, but children risk developing dependence, which is not a problem with Buspar.

---

[54] M.A. Riddle, G.A. Bernstein, E.H. Cook, H.L. Leonard, J.S. March, and J.M. Swanson. "Anxiolytics, Adrenergic Agents and Naltrexone." *Journal of the American Academy of Child and Adolescent Psychiatry* 38(5): 546–556 (1999).

[55] Wilens, op. cit., 228–231.

Buspar also has some effects on ADHD and depression. Both Buspar and benzodiazepine side effects are mild and include drowsiness and decreased mental clarity. Buspar may also reduce inhibitions.

In the abstract of a recent major review of the literature cited above, the authors conclude "that there are virtually no controlled data that support the efficacy of most of these drugs for the treatment of psychiatric disorders in children and adolescents is both surprising and unfortunate. For some drugs, e.g. buspirone and guanfacine, this is because no controlled studies have been carried out in children and/or adolescents. For other drugs, e.g. clonidine and naltrexone, most of the placebo controlled studies have failed to demonstrate efficacy."[56]

Is It Crazy to Use Antipsychotics for Children?

Antipsychotic drugs are best reserved for cases of actual psychosis, for which they are quite effective. They are increasingly used, however, as treatments of last resort for children with mood instability, tic disorders, or self-injurious and aggressive behavior who do not respond sufficiently to other medications. These drugs work by blocking dopamine receptors. The older generation of drugs is typified by Haldol (haloperidol), Mellararil (thioridazine), Navane (thiothixene), and Stelazine (trifluoperazine). The newer generation, which includes Risperidal, Seraquel, and Zyprexa, has similar but less frequent side effects.

The risk/benefit ratio must be carefully examined for these medications before they are given to a child or

---

[56] Wilens, op. cit., 236.

adolescent. They can have significant and serious short-term side effects such as dizziness, decongestion, and blurred vision. The more long-term liabilities include tardive dyskinesia (a disorder of involuntary movements) and other extrapyramidal effects (outside the brain) on muscle groups that cause spasm, rolling eyes and restlessness, and Parkinson-like symptoms of slowing, tremor, tenseness, and a masked face.[57] Side effects like these are only worth the risk in severe cases that do not respond to milder treatment. We believe that homeopathic medicine offers a much gentler alternative with far less risk.

A Safer Alternative to Psychiatric Drugs for Children

Based on our clinical experience and the reported cases of other homeopathic physicians, we believe that homeopathy offers an effective alternative to stimulants, antidepressants and other psychotropic drugs in the treatment of ADHD. We are convinced that our clinical results, even more than our experience or opinions, speak for themselves. If even a small percentage of children currently taking stimulants or other medications can enjoy instead the long-term, deep-acting benefits of homeopathy, this book will have served its purpose. For those of you who are satisfied with having your children on psychiatric medications, we are not trying to prove you wrong. For those of you who are skeptical of homeopathy or of any other alternative, please read this book in its entirety before making your decision.

---

[57] Wilens, op. cit., 346.

For those of you who are unwilling to even consider any treatment that has not been proven by scientific research, we can offer only one such study on
ADHD, a double-blind partial crossover study published
in 1997 in the British Homeopathic Journal. The study
showed positive results for homeopathic treatment of
ADHD as compared with placebo controls.[58] We realize
that this research, though promising, is only the beginning. More studies will need to be done, as funding and
institutional support for homeopathic research become
more available. (Other studies on homeopathic medicine in general and for other non-psychiatric conditions
may be found in the next chapter.)

[58] J. Lamont. "Homeopathic Treatment of Attention Deficit Hyperactivity Disorder." *British Homeopathic Journal* 86: 10,196-200 (1997).

6

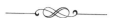

Different Strokes for Different Folks
What Parents and Kids Say About Drugs for ADHD

A Matter of Mixed Reactions

Some children and adolescents, and their parents, are satisfied using Ritalin for ADHD. Some are not. Some doubt that they could manage in their day-to-day lives if it weren't for the aid of stimulant drugs, while others complain of the side effects or parents lament that their stimulant-medicated children are no longer the vibrant kids they once knew. And then there are kids that are simply oblivious to how they feel or function, whether they are taking conventional medications, homeopathic medicine, or receiving no treatment at all. They are the "I'm fine. No problem!" kids. Many kids with ADHD already feel stigmatized because they must be in special classes or resource rooms or are slower to catch on in class. The added embarrassment of having to be present and accounted for in the medication lineup makes them feel even worse. We saw one self-conscious girl recently who wanted nothing more than to fit in and be normal. Not only did she have to stand in line for Ritalin, but also the special-education classes in which she was placed were held in a trailer apart from all of the other classrooms. She could no longer engage in friendly chitchat with her peers as they passed in the mainstream hallway, so to speak. Instead, she lowered her head in shame as she paraded past all of the normal classrooms on her way to "the trailer." Her mom couldn't believe the insensitivity of whoever designed that particular setup.

The following reactions are of children medicated with Ritalin for ADHD whom we have treated with homeopathic medicine, and of their parents. We have tried to include varying points of view, though most of the patients we have quoted are biased in the sense that they sought a more natural alternative to stimulant medication.

"I Still Have That Prescription in My Purse"

"When Michael started having problems in school and the teachers and counselors suggested ADHD, we took him to his regular pediatrician. After a forty-five-minute examination, the doctor proclaimed that he was indeed hyperactive and wrote a prescription for twenty milligrams of Ritalin every morning. I can tell you that I still have that prescription in my purse because I just couldn't believe it. We asked about diet, about allergies, about a different form of discipline. Each time the response was the same: Ritalin.

"For some reason it seems to me that our society has come to a point where everyone thinks that you just have to take a pill and whatever problem you have will get better. I just couldn't see giving my child a prescription that ultimately altered his personality. Michael has always been a kind, loving, generous, helpful child. He just doesn't sit still very well at times. I love Michael as he is and I didn't want a pill to change him."

"It Literally Saved Our Lives"

"If Rich had not been given Ritalin at age seven, I don't even care to imagine where or how bad off he would be today. It literally saved our lives! First of all, Rich's reaction to Ritalin gave us the confirmation we needed that there was indeed something physically different about him. Within fifteen minutes after receiving his first dose, we could actually witness him calming down. He could sit still, he could focus, he could carry on a real conversation. He felt good about himself and about life—not high as some people are on speed, but just 'normal' for the first time ever. His social relationships and anger were also improved.

"However, after a few months the side effects of this drug also became difficult to handle. Ritalin did not stay in Rich's system for a predictable length of time. When it wore off, he crashed. We were then given Dexedrine to take along with the Ritalin. The Dexedrine is a time-release capsule, so it was longer lasting. But, if he took it alone, it left him almost too calm. The Ritalin sort of gave him his life back. Together these medicines worked well for Rich for almost two years. Then he was diagnosed with Tourette's disorder, which manifested itself in tics and twitches. These were made worse by the Ritalin and eventually he had to discontinue the Dexedrine as well."

None of the Conventional Medications Worked

"Jared is irritable, defensive, and offends easily. He is obsessive about all kinds of things and doesn't show a lot of common sense. He doesn't think before he does things. He has a very hard time in the classroom focusing if something else is going on. He is very intense and interrupts all the time. He is easily touched. Sentimentality and rage are both very close to the surface.

"We tried Ritalin, Cylert, and Prozac. None of them worked. Ritalin made him very frantic and racing and kept him up until two in the morning on even the smallest dose. He became very weepy. With Prozac, he had absolutely no initiative. That's why we're bringing him now to you to try homeopathy." (Quotes from a mother whose child just began homeopathic treatment.)

Ritalin Rebound

"Clay, thirteen, has been on Ritalin for seven years. Because of hormonal changes during puberty, each dose only lasts three hours. What Ritalin does to Clay after he has been off the medication and goes back on is frightening—the tears, the anger. It's that chemical adjustment, like falling off a mountain. The rebound symptoms are worse than when he's off Ritalin entirely. When we tried to stop the medicine for a period of time, it took him four to six weeks to readjust. He had real problems with appetite from the Ritalin. If I wouldn't time the dose and a meal just right, he'd skip a whole meal. Now he just has less of an appetite because of the Ritalin but doesn't skip meals. Other rebound symptoms are headaches and stomachaches.

"Dexedrine also causes a rebound effect with Clay. It lasts only four to six weeks, then, if we try to increase the dosage, he becomes terribly angry and unmotivated."

When we asked Clay how he felt about taking Ritalin, he replied, "I don't like it. I have to wait to eat. I need to leave class to take my medicine and it messes up my sports because sometimes I have too much energy and other times too little."

"Ritalin Worked Really Well Sometimes— Sometimes Not"

Brad has trouble paying attention. Without Ritalin and before he was under homeopathic treatment, he became hyper. Brad had a terrible time paying attention and filtering out the environment. He was constantly asking, "What did they say?" He had no restraint. He would eat a whole pack of gum or a sack of candy in one day. He was either very sweet or very awful. There were days when he was easy to get along with and others when he became frustrated and angry, and you couldn't reason with him. He can just get higher and higher and higher. "Ritalin worked really well sometimes; sometimes not. We wanted to try a more natural treatment so that Brad would have fewer ups and downs."

Jeremy and Krissy

"Jeremy was the perfect child while he was on Ritalin. If you could package a little boy who was polite and sweet, that's how he would be. But he still had trouble concentrating in school. He wouldn't forget things, though, and he got along great with other kids. It was a nightmare when he stopped taking it for a few days or it wore off . . . he would have a rebound. After taking Ritalin for five years, Jeremy developed tics. Now, several years later, he still has them. The tics started like shivers. When the tics are bad, Jeremy is so embarrassed that he doesn't even want to go to school. We tried him on four different stimulant and antidepressant drugs but they didn't work for him. They wanted to try Prozac, but I said no. I didn't want a child of six on Prozac. I don't think I'd ever put him back on Ritalin.

"The same is true with my daughter Krissy. She developed five different side effects from Ritalin. She couldn't gain weight. She looked like a skeleton . . . like a stick figure or someone with anorexia. She was on Ritalin for three years and didn't gain weight until we took her off of it. She also chewed her nails to the quick. Nail-biting is a side effect of Ritalin in some children, you know. Krissy's anxiety level got really high from the drug, too. She would start worrying at eleven in the morning whether she would miss her school bus at three in the afternoon. She got so anxious that she laid out her toothbrush and clothes before going to bed. Sleep was another problem. While she was on Ritalin Krissy didn't want to go to sleep at night.

"We discontinued the medicine a few months ago and now we want to try homeopathy since it has helped her brother."

"It's Not the Real You. It's a Fake Person"

Not all children with ADHD feel better on Ritalin. John Merrow interviewed four teenagers who clearly did not

want to continue taking Ritalin.[59] They complained,
"It's not the real you. It's a fake person. It's totally not
me." One of the boys had discontinued the medication
by his own choice. A second had been on Ritalin for
seven years and begged his parents not to make him take
it, but one of his teachers would not allow him in her
classroom unless he had a note signed by the school
nurse that he had received his Ritalin at school that day.
The boys complained of dizziness, stomach upset, inability to sleep, a buzzed feeling, and appetite loss as a
result of taking Ritalin.

What Researchers Have Discovered

A study conducted nearly twenty years ago, entitled
"How Do Hyperactive Children Feel About Taking Stimulants and Will They Tell The Doctor?", found that 42
percent of children disliked taking Ritalin and avoided
doing so when possible, while 30 percent enjoyed it,
and another 30 percent didn't care one way or the
other.[60] Some parents in the program found their kids
easy to medicate; others had to practically chase down
their kids to make the medicine go down. This fact re-
minds us of Emmanuel, a sneaky, defiant young man
whom we treated for ADHD and conduct disorder.
Manny didn't hesitate to buck authority or to hide his
Ritalin pills under the rug for two years. The crime remained undiscovered until his mother happened to pull
up the carpet. She had to admit that, when he *was* actu-

[59] The Merrow Report, op. cit.

[60] Ester Sleator, Rina Ullmann, and Alice von Neumann, "How Do
Hyperactive Children Feel About Taking Stimulants and Will They
Tell the Doctor?" *Clinical Pediatrics* 21: 474–479 (1982).

ally taking his Ritalin, he wasn't the same Manny she knew before he was medicated. He obviously took the matter into his own hands to retain his personality and independence.

A second study revealed, as we noted, that children who were forced to receive more than one dose of Ritalin at school were unhappier, and perhaps more humiliated, than those on the sustained-release form of the drug.[61]

It is interesting to note that kids on Ritalin have a greater tendency to attribute improvements in their performance to their own efforts, rather than to the enhanced benefits of the drug, while blaming their inadequacies on not having taken medication.[62] This brings into play the idea of drug dependence. We have observed that there is a particular type of I'll-do-it-my-way type of child that may be resistant to taking any medications for ADHD, whether conventional or homeopathic. They are absolutely convinced that whatever they do must be a result of their natural, unmedicated selves. Given how gentle and harmless we and others have found homeopathy to be, this can sometimes be frustrating, however a number of parents may place the ultimate decision in the hands of the child unless the behavior or school performance is truly over-the-top. This issue is more likely to arise in adolescents who are exploring the boundaries of their independence and self-determination or may simply refuse to do anything their parents want them to do.

[61] Jennifer Bowen, Terrace Fenton, and Leonar Rappaport, "Stimulant Medication and Attention-Deficit Hyperactivity Disorder: The Child's Perspective," *American Journal of Diseases in Children* 145: 291–295 (1991).
[62] Lawrence Diller, op. cit., 260.

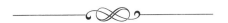

PART TWO

Homeopathy: A Whole Child Approach

7

All About Homeopathy
Natural Medicine That Works

What Is Homeopathic Medicine?

Homeopathy is a unique form of medicine that comes from different roots than does conventional medicine. It was developed as a response to the so-called "heroic" healing methods of eighteenth-century Europe—and later the United States—that included the use of toxic substances such as mercury and arsenic in large doses, as well as purging, vomiting, bloodletting, and leeches. Samuel Hahnemann (1755–1843), a brilliant German physician, chemist, and medical translator, was a harsh critic of the methods of his day and worked very hard to find a rational alternative that followed the healing principles of nature. Fluent in at least seven languages, Hahnemann extensively studied the ancient and current medical literature to discover what he believed to be the true principles of healing.

Two Paradoxes

Hahnemann's two principal discoveries were termed the "Law of Similars" and the idea of using microdoses, extremely tiny doses of medicine, to stimulate the body's ability to heal itself. Both of these discoveries are inherently paradoxical. The Law of Similars states that a substance from nature that has the ability to *cause* a set of symptoms in a healthy person can *cure* those same symptoms in a sick person. The substance that produces the most similar symptoms will heal most effectively. Using toxic or poisonous substances for healing is paradoxical, but Hahnemann found them to work quite effectively when used in the right way. Depending on how you use them, poisons kill or poisons cure.

Hahnemann first discovered the Law of Similars during an experiment to discover why quinine (the active substance in today's conventional antimalarial drugs), extracted from Peruvian Cinchona bark, cured malaria. The accepted explanation that it cured because it was bitter did not satisfy Hahnemann because he was aware of many other bitter herbs that did not cure malaria. Hahnemann himself took repeated doses of the extract to see what would happen. He developed periodic chills and fever, common symptoms of malaria. He reasoned that the bark was effective in treating malaria because it could produce symptoms similar to the disease.

He went on to test more than 100 substances on himself and his students to discover what symptoms they would produce. Applying the results of his findings in his clinical practice, he found that this new form of medicine successfully treated a significant number of patients with acute and chronic diseases that up to that time had been considered incurable.

Many physicians of Hahnemann's time were favorably impressed with his ideas and experiments, and especially with his clinical results in treating mental and emotional, as well as physical, illnesses. The use of homeopathy spread rapidly in the early nineteenth century and became renowned for its effectiveness in treating such epidemic diseases as cholera, malaria, typhoid, yellow fever, and scarlet fever.

Weaker Is Stronger

To accomplish healing without significant side effects, Hahnemann realized that the dose of whatever substance he administered must be very small. Large doses were effective based on the Law of Similars, but their toxic side effects made them less appealing as medicines. He created small doses by repeatedly diluting the original substance in a water and alcohol mixture until it was too weak to be toxic and was thus a safe, effective medicine. Hahnemann found, however, that if he diluted the medicines too much, they lost their effectiveness. He learned to retain the effectiveness of the medicine and to actually make it stronger by performing *succussion* (a process of shaking the medicine to evenly distribute the liquid). He called the combined process of serial dilution and succussion *potentization.*

Homeopaths commonly use medicines made with 30, 200, 1,000, or 10,000 dilutions, far exceeding the point at which molecules of the original substance should remain in the solution. How is this possible? No one really knows how the information pattern in homeopathic medicines persists during dilution beyond the disappearance of the physical molecules of the original substance. This has caused skepticism and prejudice about homeopathy in scientific circles, because the mechanism that preserves the pattern through the potentization process is unknown. Theories have been suggested that polarized molecules such as those in alcohol or water are capable of forming liquid crystals that "remember" the pattern of the original substance.

Homeopathic medicines produce very different effects depending on the original substance from which they were derived. Even at very high dilution factors, each medicine retains its unique characteristics and the ability to dramatically affect people's health. Some factor must persist at high dilutions, which is responsible for the clinical success of homeopathic medicines. We look forward to additional scientific research that will confirm precisely how homeopathy works. A recently published book, *Homeopathy: A Frontier in Medical Science,* gives a good review of these controversial issues, as well as current research on homeopathic medicine.[1]

Is There Research on Homeopathy?

In research using common medical conditions, double-blind clinical studies have shown the effectiveness of homeopathic medicine as compared with a placebo. The most recent major review of the literature on the effectiveness of homeopathic medicine was a 1997 state-of-the-art meta-analysis published in the *Lancet.*[2] Of the 186 studies analyzed, 89 fit the criteria for the meta-analysis. In those studies, homeopathic medicines had a 2.45 times greater effect than placebo. A 1991 review of more than one hundred homeopathic research studies

[1] Paolo Bellavite and Andrea Signorini, *Homeopathy: A Frontier in Medical Science* (Berkeley: North Atlantic, 1995).

[2] K. Linde, N. Clausius, G. Ramirez, *et al.,* "Are the Clinical Effects of Homoeopathy Placebo Effects? A Meta-analysis of Placebo-Controlled Trials," *The Lancet* 350: 834–843 (1997).

published between 1966 and 1990 showed that homeopathy showed positive results in 76 percent of the studies in conditions that included infections, digestive disorders, influenza, hay fever, rheumatoid arthritis, fibromyalgia, recovery from surgery, and psychological problems. The authors concluded that although they could not account for the positive results, the results did warrant further research using better methodology.[3] A study published in 1994 by the peer-reviewed journal *Pediatrics,* by Jennifer Jacobs, M.D., and associates, demonstrated homeopathy's effectiveness in pediatric diarrhea in Nicaragua.[4] In another major study, also published in the British journal *The Lancet* in 1994, Scottish researcher David Taylor Reilly and his associates found that 82 percent of asthma sufferers who were treated with homeopathic dilutions of their main allergens improved significantly, compared to the 38 percent improvement in the placebo control group.[5]

Unfortunately, researchers have not been able to study the effects of homeopathic treatment on ADHD because of lack of funding, except in one case. The Lamont study, mentioned in the previous chapter, is the one piece of homeopathic research to date on children with ADHD. Lamont used a single homeopathic medicine approach, as we recommend in this book, on forty-three children with ADHD. His statistically significant results corroborated that homeopathic treatment is superior to

---

[3] J. Kleijnan, P. Knipschild, and G. ter Riet, "Clinical Trials of Homeopathy," *British Medical Journal* 302: 316–323 (1991).

[4] L. Jacobs, M. Jimenez, S. Gloyd, and D. Crothers, "Treatment of Acute Childhood Diarrhea with Homeopathic Medicine: A Randomized Clinical Trial in Nicaragua," *Pediatrics* 94(5): 719–725 (1994).

[5] David Reilly, Morag Taylor, Neil Beattie, *et al.,* "Is Evidence for Homeopathy Reproducible?" *The Lancet* 344: 1601–1606 (1994).

placebo.[6] Homeopaths have always, and continue to, base their evidence for the effectiveness of homeopathy on clinical results with many patients. These results are shared in professional homeopathic journals and case conferences. It is unfortunate that the scientific community still holds double-blind, placebo-controlled research as the only measure of the validity of any method of treatment because clinical evidence of the effectiveness of homeopathic treatment of ADHD speaks for itself.

Homeopathy Remains Controversial Among Mainstream Thinkers

It may initially be difficult to grasp the idea of homeopathy; that substances that cause symptoms can also cure them, and that tiny doses work even if they are diluted past the point where the substance physically disappears. Some people encountering these facts about homeopathy think that they cannot possibly be correct. How, then, does one explain how homeopathic medicines have repeatedly demonstrated positive clinical results in controlled studies? That the basis for homeopathy is unknown should not lead to discounting it, but to a greater effort to understand it. Unfortunately, conventional medical science has not yet made an unbiased investigation of homeopathy, mostly due to prejudice and fear of academic ridicule for investigating a taboo subject. Those physicians and scientists who do investigate homeopathy with an open mind often change from critics to proponents.

[6] John Lamont, "Homeopathic Treatment of Attention Deficit Hyperactivity Disorder." *British Homeopathic Journal* 86(10): 196–200 (1997).

What Makes Homeopathy Unique?

Homeopathy is very different from other forms of medicine. Conventional medicine often treats conditions with various kinds of drugs, which may interact negatively with each other, or cause complex combinations of side effects. Homeopathy uses only a single medicine because of the single principle that guides homeopathic practice, the Law of Similars.

The challenge in homeopathy is to pick the one substance from nature that truly matches the patient's symptoms. Rather than giving many different drugs to a patient, a homeopath gives only a single natural medicine that is individualized according to the patient's pattern of symptoms. Homeopaths treat the *patient,* not the disease. This means that ten patients with ADHD may need ten different homeopathic medicines. Their individual differences are what lead the homeopath to choose a particular medicine that can help each of them lead a happier, better adjusted, more productive life. The homeopathic medicine must match the patient's symptom pattern or picture to be effective. When the match is made well and the prescription is correct, the patient's condition will markedly improve—physically, mentally, and emotionally.

Although homeopathic medicines are made from substances that can cause symptoms if given too frequently or in too large a dose, the microdoses used in homeopathic treatment are extremely safe. They are largely free from side effects. Some patients may experience a brief initial worsening of their symptoms before improving, which may last from few hours to a week or more. Rarely, the patient may briefly experience new symptoms that belong to the medicine if the dosage is too frequent, but these will usually go away readily when the medicine is stopped.

From Tarantulas to Platinum

Homeopathic medicines come from all over the world and from extremely diverse substances. Virtually any naturally occurring substance can be used as a homeopathic medicine. Medicines are made from all three kingdoms: animal, plant, and mineral. Poisonous plants, such as digitalis and *Agaricus muscaria* (toxic mushrooms); venom from snakes and spiders, such as rattlesnake and tarantula; milk of mammals, such as humans, dogs, and dolphins; and mineral elements and their salts, such as platinum, table salt, and sulphur are all used as homeopathic medicines. Hidden in each of these substances is a unique pattern of the symptoms people develop when they become ill. A few of the homeopathic medicines that have been used successfully for ADHD include the substance secreted by the tarantula spider *(Tarentula hispanica),* white hellebore *(Veratrum album),* datura stramonium *(Stramonium),* deadly nightshade *(Belladonna),* iodide of arsenic *(Arsenicum iodatum),* zinc *(Zincum metallicum),* and silver nitrate *(Argentum nitricum).* Many other homeopathic medicines can also be used depending on the unique symptoms of the patient.

The secrets of the substances used in homeopathy are unlocked by experiments called *provings,* which were initially done by Hahnemann and his students on healthy volunteers, including themselves. In a proving, a substance unknown to the participants or *provers* is given in either a crude dose if its toxicity is not too great or in a homeopathic dilution until the provers begin to develop symptoms. Provers record whatever happens to them physically, mentally, and emotionally during the experiment. These records are carefully analyzed to determine the symptoms that the particular substance can produce and ultimately cure when made into a potentized homeopathic medicine.

Provings done on the same substance in different parts of the world often yield remarkably similar results, demonstrating the universality of the Law of Similars. All provers do not respond identically to a given substance. Some are more susceptible, others less so. One prover may respond with more physical symptoms, while another may manifest emotional or mental problems. With a large enough group, however, the full picture of the substance emerges. Provers often report personal health benefits from participating in the proving.

Provings are still being done today. Recent provings have used chocolate, hydrogen, dolphin's and lion's milks, lavender, scorpion, tungsten, eagle's blood, neon, plutonium, and other sources, allowing these diverse substances to be used effectively as homeopathic medicines.

Regulation and Availability of Homeopathic Medicines

The Food and Drug Administration (FDA) regulates homeopathic medicines as over-the-counter (OTC) drugs. According to information from the American Homeopathic Pharmaceutical Association in Valley Forge, Pennsylvania, sales of homeopathic medicines are currently increasing at a rate of about 20 percent per year. Homeopathic pharmacies must follow rigid guidelines established by the *Homeopathic Pharmacopoeia of the*

United States. Some of these medicines are available over the counter in pharmacies or health food stores. Others can only be obtained by licensed medical practitioners. The doses available over the counter are often considerably lower than would be used by a homeopathic physician in the case of ADHD. The medicines referred to in this book are always single-substance preparations, as opposed to combination homeopathic medicines that are available to treat colds, flus, and other acute conditions if one is not under the care of a homeopath.

Homeopathy Throughout the World

Homeopathy is only beginning to be rediscovered in the United States. A 1993 study published in the *New England Journal of Medicine* revealed that one-third of all Americans are using some form of alternative medicine and that, in 1990, two and a half million Americans used homeopathy and made nearly five million visits to homeopathic practitioners.[7]

In India, England, France, Germany, Mexico, and South America, homeopathic medicine is widely practiced. The royal family in England has used and supported homeopathy extensively since 1830. More than twenty homeopathic schools or part-time courses flourish in England, including a course for medical doctors at the Royal London Homeopathic Hospital. The Society of Homeopaths maintains a registry of homeopathic practitioners, and 42 percent of British family practi-

---

[7] David M. Eisenberg, Ronald C. Kessler, Cindy Foster, *et al.,* "Unconventional Medicine in the United States," *New England Journal of Medicine* 328(4): 146–252 (1993).

tioners refer to homeopaths.[8] More than 11,000 French physicians use homeopathic medicines, which are dispensed by more than 20,000 pharmacies.[9] Thirty-six percent of French citizens have been treated homeopathically.[10] Homeopathic treatment is reimbursed through the national health care system in France and some other European countries. Excellent postgraduate homeopathic courses are offered widely throughout Europe. India has more than 120 homeopathic medical colleges, and more than 100,000 homeopathic practitioners, a legacy of the British Raj.[11] The United States is behind the times in its acceptance of homeopathy.

[8] Richard Wharton and George Lewith, "Complementary Medicine and the General Practitioner," *British Medical Journal* 292: 1498–1500 (1986).

[9] Dana Ullman, *Discovering Homeopathy-Medicine for the 21st Century* (Berkeley: North Atlantic Books, 1988), 48.

[10] Dana Ullman, *The Consumer's Guide to Homeopathy* (New York: Tarcher/Putnam, 1996), 36.

[11] Ibid., 39.

8

A Better Answer Than Ritalin
Homeopathy Is a Highly Effective Treatment for ADHD

What if you heard about a way to treat ADHD without drugs, in fact not just ADHD, but *all* of your child's problems, including her headaches and asthma? A method that would value all that is special and creative about your child while simultaneously recognizing the specific ways in which she could change for the better? A type of natural medicine that could help your child learn more easily and improve her grades, be less bouncy and off-the-wall, and have more friends and feel lots better about herself? Would you listen? You bet. That's exactly what homeopathy offers your child, and it's why so many parents who are listening are choosing homeopathy over conventional medication to help their children with ADHD and other problems.

Each child or adult you will read about in this book has a story, perhaps much like that of your own child. In fact, it may even seem as if we were writing about *your* child. However, in truth, each child is distinctive and deserves to be listened to, understood, and treated in an individualized way. Homeopaths have the time and inclination to explore your child in depth. To a homeopath, your child is not a body or a diagnosis, but a very special person whose life can be brought into balance and very much changed for the better.

Why Choose Homeopathy Over Conventional Medicine for ADHD?

- Homeopathy works. This approach has been very successful with many thousands of children with ADHD and other behavioral and learning problems.
- Simply put, homeopathy makes sense.
- Homeopathy is safe, natural, and lacks the side effects of conventional medicine. Homeopathic medicines never suppress a child's normal growth and development. In fact, many children experience a growth spurt after beginning homeopathic treatment. Nor does homeopathy cause such side effects as anxiety, appetite suppression, insomnia, or tics, or have a rebound effect as can Ritalin.
- A standard dose of Ritalin, unless it is slow release, lasts only about four hours. One dose of the correct

The Pros of Homeopathic Treatment of ADHD

- Treats the whole person at the root of the problem
- Considered safe, without the side effects of Ritalin and other medications
- Uses natural, nontoxic medicines
- Treats each person as an individual
- Heals physical as well as mental and emotional symptoms
- Lasts for months or years rather than hours
- Medicine is inexpensive
- Treatment is cost-effective

homeopathic medicine often lasts four to six months or longer.

- Homeopathic medicines are very inexpensive compared with Ritalin and other conventional drugs for ADHD. The only significant cost of homeopathic treatment is office visits. Once your child has responded well to homeopathy, appointments are infrequent.
- Homeopathy treats the whole person. Not only do learning and behavioral problems improve, so do most or all of the other physical, mental, and emotional complaints of the person. Conventional medication for ADHD works only on specific learning and behavioral problems. Sally Smith, a parent of an ADHD child formerly on Ritalin, describes this phenomenon by holding up a ruler and pointing to the one-inch mark: "Ritalin makes you available to learn. You and your parents and teachers have to work on all the rest."[12]
- Homeopathy will not make a child depressed or dull. Parents sometimes complain that, although stimulant and antidepressant medications have eliminated some of the more severe problem behaviors, their children's spirits seem dampened and they are no longer themselves.
- Homeopathic medicines are generally given infrequently and over limited periods of time. Many physicians prescribe Ritalin and other medications for life.

What Can You Expect from Homeopathic Treatment of Your Child with ADHD?

You can expect at least a 70 percent improvement, over time, in the following:

---

[12] "Mother's Little Helper," *Newsweek,* March 18, 1996, 50–56.

- behavior at home and at school
- ability to concentrate
- grades
- impulsivity
- restlessness
- ability to make friends
- socially appropriate behavior
- mood
- relationships with the rest of the family
- self-esteem
- confidence
- independence
- physical health complaints
- overall health
- immunity

These changes begin within two to five weeks after taking the correct homeopathic medicine, but the improvement continues and stabilizes. That is why it is essential to continue homeopathic treatment for at least one to two years. Even though very positive changes can take place rapidly, the most profound effects of homeopathy result from continuing for a period of years, although the appointments are likely to be less and less frequent, eventually only a couple of times a year.

Can Homeopathy Be Used Along with or Instead of Conventional Medicine?

Many of the children that we treat are on Ritalin or other medications when they begin homeopathic treatment. The approach that we have found to be most effective, gentle, and to satisfy everyone concerned, is to continue the medication until we find the correct medicine for the child. When this is evident, and the child's problems are considerably better, then the parents can consult with the prescribing physician concerning discontinuing or tapering off the conventional medications. In cases where the child derives no benefit at all from the conventional medicine, the prescribing physician and patient generally agree to discontinue it and, instead, and to begin homeopathic care. If the Ritalin or other drug is working, but the side effects are disturbing, or if you do not like the idea of having your child continue to take stimulants or other medications over time, be honest with your doctor about your desire to seek an alternative. Some parents prefer to keep their children on both conventional and homeopathic medicine, often as a type of insurance policy that their children will succeed, however once the right homeopathic medicine has been prescribed, the conventional drugs are usually not necessary.

Homeopathy Instead of Stimulants

The following cases describe two of many children we have treated with homeopathy who have been able to discontinue conventional medications.

"He Goes After Life with Gusto"   Rajiv's mom described him as "eleven going on twenty." His parents had found Rajiv's behavior challenging early on, leading them to attend parenting classes when he was four years old. Headstrong and opinionated, Rajiv was a chief. To his credit, he had great ideas, but didn't always know how to pull them off gracefully. Though very adept verbally, Rajiv had trouble with reading, writing, and drawing pictures. As he got older, even though reading continued to be difficult for him, he was drawn to technical magazines such as *Popular Mechanics*.

Defiant, he rarely complied when his parents routinely told him to do something. Unless his timing and theirs coincided, they were out of luck. Rajiv had the habit of placing conditions on even the simplest requests made of him. According to his parents, he was a Bill Gates-type-of kid—a visionary who didn't much care about conforming to the social norm. He took after his dad, "a computer nut," who was not fond of being shown how to do things. Eccentric in a variety of ways, Rajiv enjoyed gardening, cooking, and growing herbs. Whether his hair was combed or his teeth were brushed were not of major concern to him.

Rajiv was taking 20 milligrams of slow-release Ritalin morning and afternoon. We prescribed *Sulphur*, a common homeopathic medicine for intelligent, eccentric, science- and computer-oriented kids who may be oblivious to hygiene and social graces. Six weeks later his parents gave a positive report: Rajiv was a good 70 percent "more mellow." More cooperative, he was less insistent on doing things his way, managed quite well at camp, and responded with, "Sure dad, I'll do it" for the first time ever. His parents were able to discontinue the Ritalin, with the encouragement of his psychiatrist, and he has never again needed it.

Now, one year later, Rajiv says he is glad that he no longer takes Ritalin. He is happier in general, more responsible, and doing better in school; his mom estimated the overall improvement at 80 percent. She confided, "When people asks me how homeopathy has helped my son so much, I tell them, 'Hey, I can't tell you *how* it works. It just does.'"

"A Troublemaker with a Heart of Gold" Regan, fourteen years old, had been a problem child since the age of two. His mother was hospitalized for three months prior to his birth because of a threatened premature delivery. She was miserable with morning sickness during the entire pregnancy. As a young child, Regan never walked but sprinted. He hit, kicked, spat, and jumped at a very early age. His father was also hyperactive.

The child was bright, with a good sense of humor and a heart of gold, but he was a real troublemaker. He laughed over his constantly impulsive behavior. He clowned, laughed, fiddled, and chewed gum in his classroom. Regan dismantled his school counselor's typewriter, for which he had to wash dishes. He loved to be the center of attention. Regan often got into trouble with his dad because of his lying.

Regan was very unhappy with himself. He tried to overdose on pills following an argument with his parents. During that argument Regan smashed his stereo speakers and pulled out his hair. When he flew into a rage, he turned into a wild man and didn't know what he was doing." Following hospitalization on a children's psychiatric ward, Regan was given an antipsychotic medication along with two tranquilizers. Previously he had taken Ritalin for a year and a half, along with Cylert and two antidepressants. He still had significant behavioral problems.

Regan had an ordinary side, too. He described himself as "a regular kid on the move." He liked to ride his bike fast, to climb, and to build and dismantle things. In fact, he had taken apart fifteen bikes. He enjoyed seeing his friends and meeting girls. He especially loved rap music; he found it so relaxing that it could put him to sleep. Regan had a preference for gang movies.

We treated Regan with *Tarentula*. At his follow-up visit after four months of treatment, he and his mother reported that his sleep was more restful and that, overall, he felt much more relaxed. Feeling calmer resulted in Regan being able to concentrate much better at school. His grades improved from Fs to As, Bs, and Cs. Regan's handwriting was now quite legible. He had very few problems in class and no more suspensions, which had not been mentioned initially. His fidgeting and nervousness had decreased markedly. His sleep had also improved. In coordination with his psychiatrist, the family had eliminated the antipsychotic medication and decreased his antidepressants. He's continued to respond well to homeopathic treatment, and over time the antidepressants were also discontinued.

Regan shared, "I've been fine. I do my work and keep my nose clean. I don't listen to rap music so much. I haven't gotten mad at all. I'm not even lying."

What If My Doctor Does Not Believe in Homeopathy?

From the time that homeopathic medicine was first brought to this country in the early 1800s, many medical doctors have remained skeptical about its efficacy and claims. Homeopathic philosophy is very different from what is taught in conventional medical schools. Your doctor may not know the difference between homeopathy and other forms of natural medicine and think that homeopathy has the same side effects as some herbs, which is definitely not true. With the growing interest in homeopathic medicine and with the disillusionment about the side effects and short-term benefits of much of modern medical treatment, some conventional doctors are opening their minds to homeopathy and even incorporating homeopathy into their conventional practices or referring to other homeopathic practitioners. We receive many referrals from physicians and other health care practitioners.

If your physician or your child's physician is adamantly opposed to your trying homeopathy, you can try to educate him about its benefits or find a physician who is more supportive of your freedom of choice. Homeopathic practitioners are generally happy to educate conventional physicians about homeopathic philosophy and treatment. Even a skeptical person may be convinced of the possible benefits of homeopathy through reading case studies, attending a homeopathic case conference, or seeing the results of successful homeopathic treatment.

What to Avoid During Homeopathic Treatment

Certain substances and exposures consistently interfere with homeopathic treatment. Most practitioners will advise you to avoid the following substances or objects: coffee, eucalyptus, camphor, menthol, recreational drugs, and electric blankets. You will be asked to avoid using topical medications such as topical steroids, antibiotics, antifungals, and to use oral antibiotics and cortisone products only after consulting your homeopath, except in cases of emergency. Acupuncture, although a very effective form of medicine, is not recommended during homeopathic treatment. Nor are other treatments, which are prescribed to remove specific symptoms without treating the whole person. Homeopathic practitioners may differ in their advice on what to avoid.

Your Responsibilities as a Homeopathic Patient

If you want to maximize the chances that you or your child will benefit from homeopathy, you need to:

- continue homeopathic treatment for at least one year before deciding to try another approach;
- provide thorough and honest information to your homeopath;
- inform him or her of any medications that your child is taking and to give a clear picture of what your child is like *without* any medications;
- avoid those substances that can interfere with homeopathic treatment;
- keep scheduled appointments; and
- inform the homeopath of any significant changes in your health during the course of homeopathic treatment.

The Limitations of Homeopathic Treatment

Homeopathic treatment is not for everyone. The following are factors that prevent a person from being a good candidate for homeopathic treatment.

- Some children, particularly teenagers, can be so opposed to anything their parents recommend that they will sabotage homeopathic treatment, either by refusing to go to appointments or take the medicines or by intentionally using substances that interfere with homeopathic treatment.
- Both parents need to be committed to giving homeopathy a chance for at least a year.
- Some children and adolescents have such severe behavioral problems that they need to be in an institution, such as a jail or drug or alcohol treatment center, rather than receiving outpatient treatment
- Some individuals are unwilling to avoid those substances that interfere with homeopathic treatment, such as coffee or recreational drugs.

- Both you and your child need to have patience in evaluating the effect of each homeopathic medicine.

Why Not Treat Yourself or Your Family?

As you read through the cases in this book, you will probably think of someone you know who may have a very similar cluster of symptoms. You may even be tempted to try to find the medicines mentioned in this book and administer them yourself. Don't even think of it!

Although it *is* possible to treat yourself and your family successfully with homeopathy for many first-aid and acute problems, ADHD and the other conditions covered in this book are *not* acute.

These are chronic states and need to be handled much more carefully. There are over 2,000 homeopathic medicines. It takes years of homeopathic study and practice to make the fine distinctions about when to prescribe which medicine. Although homeopathic medicines do not have long lists of side effects like many conventional medicines, it is possible to experience a reaction to the medicine, particularly if it is used incorrectly. IN ANY CHRONIC CONDITION, WHETHER PHYSICAL, MENTAL, OR EMOTIONAL, DO NOT TREAT YOURSELF OR YOUR CHILD. Find an experienced homeopathic practitioner. If you were considering brain surgery, you would not read a book or two, buy a set of scalpels, and start cutting. Homeopathy is just as complicated an art as neurosurgery. Just because homeopathic medicines are widely available does not mean they are easy to use. Please do not experiment on yourself or your family members for ADHD. Find an expert.

How Can I Find a Homeopath?

A growing number of health care practitioners, including naturopathic physicians (N.D.), medical doctors (M.D.), osteopathic physicians (D.O.), chiropractors (D.C.), family nurse practitioners (F.N.P.), physicians' assistants (P.A.), acupuncturists (L.A., C.A., or O.M.D.), and veterinarians (D.V.M.), practice homeopathic medicine. Some homeopaths are unlicensed. We know of no experienced homeopaths in the United States who focus solely on patients with ADHD.

The following are important criteria in selecting a homeopath to treat your child with ADHD:

- specialization or, preferably, board certification in homeopathic medicine
- practices *classical* homeopathy, which means that she spends at least one hour with new patients and half an hour for return visits, prescribes one medicine at a time then waits, and chooses the medicines by means of in-depth interviews rather than machines or muscle testing.
- if not board certified, has a minimum of 500 hours of training in classical homeopathy
- devotes a minimum of 75 percent of her practice to homeopathy
- has been in practice at least three, and preferably five, years
- has treated a number of children with ADHD

You cannot always find a homeopath in your immediate area, or even your state. You are likely to find much better results with an experienced homeopath, even if you need to travel or do your homeopathic consultations by telephone. Because homeopaths are specialists and prescriptions are based on interviews, a local physician can perform physical examinations, if needed. We treat many patients by phone, though we prefer to do the initial interview in person if at all possible.

In the appendix you can find the names and addresses of organizations that publish directories of homeopathic practitioners in the United States. It is still wise to speak to the practitioner directly to make sure he or she meets the guidelines we have suggested.

9

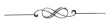

Unique Treatment for
Unique Individuals
Treating People, Not Diagnoses

There are tremendous variations in the behaviors, personalities, and characteristics of children who fall under the one diagnostic umbrella of ADHD. This diagnosis may include a violent, aggressive child who smashes doors and bites his playmates, as well as a mild-mannered, shy, well-behaved child who just can't focus. In conventional medicine, these two children will both be diagnosed with ADHD and are likely to be given Ritalin or another stimulant medication. But they are two extremely different individuals. Their diagnosis of ADHD may be the only thing these two kids have in common.

This is one of the ways in which homeopathy and orthodox medicine differ significantly. Each child, or adult, is much like a jigsaw puzzle. Once all of the pieces are assembled in their proper places, an image emerges that is distinct from other puzzles. It is the task of a homeopath to recognize that image and to match it to the corresponding image of one specific homeopathic medicine. This is accomplished by one or more in-depth interviews in which the homeopath elicits the specific behaviors, feelings, attitudes, beliefs, likes, dislikes, and preferences of the child. Also important are dreams, fears, physical symptoms, prenatal and birth history, family medical history, and eating and sleeping habits. The intent is to understand the child from the inside out. This is a completely different type of interview from the kind that a psychiatrist or psychologist might perform to diagnose ADHD. The homeopath is not interested in labels, but in what makes the child tick, how he thinks about himself, and how he approaches the world.

It is the unusual symptoms or characteristics, rather than those that are common among most children with ADHD, that are the greatest aids in finding the correct homeopathic medicine. It is typical for kids to love pizza and ice cream, but much rarer for a child to rave about artichoke hearts or spinach soufflé or to love drinking vinegar. We saw a child recently who was fixated on tornadoes and hurricanes. He loved their whirling motion and twirled his hands incessantly to mimic this motion. That is odd. Many kids blow their allowance on candy and video games, but we treated one adolescent who diligently saved her money to donate to a save-the-whales foundation. This is out of the ordinary in our society. It is the quirky symptoms that are much more likely to be of interest to a homeopath than the normal or common symptoms.

Perceiving the State of Each Child

Each child has a *state*. That state is the mental-emotional-physical stance that he has adopted that determines how he interacts with the rest of the world. Take Jimmy, for example, whose story we told in the introduction to this book. Jimmy had been subjected to profound neglect and abuse. His mother chased Jimmy into the bathroom repeatedly to beat him. His response: to keep moving. Even after Jimmy was long gone from his birth mother, the pattern continued—perpetual motion—even when he needed to sleep or to be attentive at school. Jim found anything and everything to keep himself busy. His hands, legs, mouth, and mind all moved incessantly. This is the state in which he became frozen in response to being physically abused by his mother. It was his best shot at protecting himself, and he continued to move long after he was safe and didn't need to escape. Another child in the same situation might respond by isolating himself in his room with his books or by writing poetry to hide and escape to a world of happiness and fantasy. A third child might mask his pain by becoming the class clown.

Just as each person has a state, each homeopathic medicine also corresponds to a state. Some medicines have states of terror, others of torment, and still others of mental paralysis or emotional anguish. There are homeopathic medicines for children who feel pursued by wild animals and for those with a desire to attack; for kids obsessed with germs on doorknobs and for those who can think of nothing but horses. For every imaginable state, there is a homeopathic medicine that matches it.

Once that particular medicine is prescribed, a shift will occur, often a dramatic one. This can take place regardless of the circumstances that brought the state into being or its duration. States are neither pleasant nor intentional. Being in balance and harmony is a much more desirable way to live.

Animal, Plant, and Mineral Types

One fascinating model that has emerged in recent years in homeopathy, introduced by Dr. Rajan Sankaran of

Bombay, India, in *The Substance of Homeopathy,* is the concept of animal, plant, and mineral personality types.[13] This model may help you grasp one way in which we think about children.

Children who need medicines made from animal sources will have characteristics and symptoms different from children who need medicines from plant or mineral sources. Once the kingdom is determined, the homeopath must still select the appropriate medicine from that kingdom. This takes considerable experience, so you can understand why it is important to seek treatment from an experienced professional rather than do your own guesswork.

Let's begin with the animal kingdom. Think of any animals, from beetles to elephants. How do they act and what issues seem important to them? The main motivation for animals is survival: food and drink, finding a mate, protecting themselves against the elements, and preventing or surviving attacks from enemies. Animals need to compete successfully to remain alive; the weakest succumb. They compete for food, mates, territory, and dominance. Animals draw attention to themselves. They often try to be more attractive and colorful than those around them.

Children with ADHD needing homeopathic medicines from animal sources are likely to be aggressive, competitive, jealous, and easily provoked. They love to be the center of attention and may do anything necessary to avoid being ignored or neglected. These kids either love or are terrified of animals and often engage in animal-like behaviors such as hitting, kicking, biting, scratching, and growling. These children and adolescents

[13] Rajan Sankaran, *The Substance of Homeopathy* (Berkeley, CA: Homeopathic Educational Services).

may feel dominated, inferior, and worthless. They will do nearly anything to avoid being excluded from their pack or group. Kids needing animal remedies may complain of ravenous, or canine, hunger and may tend toward crude, even primitive, behaviors. They often find it challenging to share the same territory with others.

Children who are plant types think and behave very differently. Plants tend to be sensitive and so are plant-like people. Plants need regular water and sunshine and healthy soil to survive. There are, of course, some extremely hardy plants, but most need favorable conditions to thrive. Plants adapt to weather changes, and children needing plant-derived homeopathic medicines aim to please, often at the expense of their own needs. These children are often gentle and mild and love nature, plants, and flowers. Once they are old enough to choose their own clothing, these children may pick out flowing garments with flower or plant designs. The kids are more likely to lack firm structure and to have changeable natures. Their feelings are often easily hurt.

ADHD kids needing plant medicines are likely to be drifty and scattered. They often have difficulty sticking with any task long enough to complete it. Highly emotional, they may make you feel as if you need to walk on eggshells when you are around them. Plant-type kids can be sensitive and affectionate, creative and whimsical, moody and inconsistent.

Now think of the mineral kingdom. What are minerals like? They are fixed, solid, and structured. Children needing mineral medicines need organization and structure to feel secure. They are very concerned with safety, security, and performance. Deliberate and determined, these children are logical, rational, and mechanical. They often speak in facts and figures, percentages, and chronological order.

Mineral-type kids with ADHD tend to be rigid and controlling. They can become nervous and insecure when out of their comfort zone. These children love to build intricate structures and to take things apart to see how they work. They may seem more stiff than spontaneous, compared to their plant or animal counterparts. These children can be very finicky about what they eat, how they dress, and what they like to do.

This animal, plant, and mineral classification is just one example of various ways in which a homeopath tries to understand what stands out about each child, which, he hopes, will lead him to select a corresponding medicine.

10

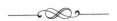

Changing Children's Lives with Homeopathy
What Parents Say About Homeopathic Treatment

Following are candid comments from some of the parents of children we have treated:

"Michael's Behavior Improved Dramatically"

"We did not want to put Michael on drugs. I was very open-minded and willing to try anything except a personality-altering drug. We racked our brains for weeks, knowing there had to be something else out there to help us. Not a drug. That's when we found you and homeopathy. After one appointment with you and a dose of homeopathic medicine, the teachers and counselors were calling me at home to find out what I had done with Michael. His behavior improved dramatically. His schoolwork turned around 180 degrees. He was able to listen and to process information. All this without Ritalin. The teachers changed their mind about Michael's diagnosis of ADHD. Any doubts or worries that I had about trying homeopathy for the first time dissipated after the calls from Michael's teacher.

Homeopathic medicine has worked wonders with him. I'm thrilled to know that there is an alternative to the traditional pop-a-pill method. Michael's success has even convinced my husband, who is studying to be a paramedic, that there may be a better way."

"Benjie Was a Wild Child"

"Benjie had always been different from other boys. Wild and aggressive, he simply could not sit still nor would he respond to anyone in authority. He was diagnosed with ADHD by teachers, our family doctor, and other professionals, and you agreed with the diagnosis. After a very thorough interview, you gave him a homeopathic medicine. Almost immediately after taking the medicine, Benjie changed. He calmed down, sat still, and would actually listen. I encourage anyone to get homeopathic help for ADHD."

"Homeopathy Has Changed Phil's Whole Attitude . . . and Ours"

"Homeopathic treatment has made a major difference in our home life and in my relationship with Phil. It's so much better. He had somehow gotten the impression from us that there was something wrong with him. Homeopathy has changed his whole attitude and ours. I can't begin to describe how much more relaxed it is around our house now. Phil can settle down and he no longer screams. He can get through the basics of the day without our needing to negotiate every little thing. I no longer worry about my son at school or in new situations nor do I pick him up from school with a sick stomach every day wondering what his teacher will tell me. A close family friend asked me what I had done to help Phil so much. She was amazed!"

"I Got My Son Back Again!"

"After our family vacation to Disneyland, I felt like I didn't know Jason anymore. It was as if someone had replaced my child with someone else. He suddenly became hateful, spit, and hit. My son even spit in his dad's face! Out of nowhere he became disrespectful and could not be satisfied. The only explanation that I can think of is that I was holding his baby sister in my lap during the trip. He started telling us that there was 'a guy in his room' and became terrified, which was totally uncharacteristic of him before the trip. Everyone told me it might be because he was sexually abused, but I knew that wasn't the case.

"I was very scared and nervous about the change in his personality. He went from sweet to spiteful overnight. His fear and aggression went away with homeopathic treatment. I felt like I got Jason back again. Often, when I look at him, I think about how I lost him temporarily. I am so thankful that I got him back! Homeopathy is so simple and safe."

"Reese's Ability to Focus Is Remarkably Better Since Homeopathy"

"I was amazed when my son told me that he couldn't concentrate at school because of the constant pictures that went through his head. They only lasted a few seconds and ranged from pleasing scenarios to scary monsters. He could not get rid of them. Within days of taking his homeopathic medicine, these images started to go away. Two weeks later they were totally gone and have not returned. The length of time that he was able to stay focused at school started increasing and he is remarkably better now than he was a year ago."

A Case Where Homeopathy Was Not Helpful

"We turned to homeopathy with our regular doctor's blessings. He had run out of answers for Rich. We tried many different homeopathic medicines over two years. We were dealing with angry, defiant behavior, hyperactivity, inability to focus, and physical tics including throat clearing and spitting. We found some medicines that did wonders with the angry, defiant behavior and hyperactivity, but the tics were still a problem. Or we found something that helped the tics, but not his other behaviors. Due to the severity of his symptoms and how profoundly they affected his daily life, especially in junior high school, we finally took him to a Tourette's disorder research specialist in California. He is now on a combination of drugs and is doing considerably better. I still believe that if Rich had more time and less pressing circumstances in his life, his homeopathic doctor could have found a medicine to meet his needs. Dr. Reichenberg-Ullman certainly found one for me, Rich's mom, that changed my life for the better and helped me cope with living with a child with ADHD and Tourette's disorder."

"Before Homeopathy He Drew Sharks. Now He Draws Funny Cartoon Characters"

"Jay is introverted and shy by nature, yet can play very cooperatively with other children. He can become angry quickly, with verbal outbursts. After his little sister was born, Jay developed recurring impetigo. He fell into the position of a silent middle child. Upon being excluded by the other children at school, Jay admitted that he felt terrible and was contemplating what it would be like to kill himself. He repeated this despairing statement on four separate occasions. An artistic young man, Jay began to draw unsuspecting swimmers being devoured by ferocious sharks.

"After being treated homeopathically, Jay's sweet personality returned and was nicer to his sister again. His impetigo cleared up. Jay stopped drawing sharks and began drawing cartoons or comical figures. We moved him to a new school where he made many friends and was elected class president. Recently Jay remarked, 'I don't let it bother me anymore when people put me down. I just go on with what I'm doing. It doesn't hurt my feelings like it did before.'"

"He's Not in Special Help Classes Anymore"

"Ray has come a long way since beginning homeopathy. He had lots of learning problems in the past that, over time, affected his self-esteem. Ray is now doing much better at school; his grades in English have come up from D's and F's to B's. He no longer attends special help classes, which thrills him as much as it does us!"

No More Ear Problems or Defiance

"I think you already know that I think homeopathy is wonderful. I first came to you with both of the girls two and a half years ago. Allie had ear infections, which her pediatrician had treated with many different courses of antibiotics. I decided that was too many drugs for a toddler, so I found you. You gave Allie homeopathic medicine for ear infections and she's never had one since. I remember that she was two years old when we first saw you and she always had a fear of dogs. Ever since that first medicine you gave her, I haven't been able to keep her away from them. Every time she sees a dog now, she asks about it. It's amazing.

"As far as disposition, Allie has been a challenge. When she has had bouts of being difficult to get along with and uncooperative, fussy, clingy, and doesn't want to do what she's asked, you've given her medicines that have really helped. She's become more receptive and open and cooperative and much more enjoyable to associate with. She also had a bad, recurrent cough that you have treated successfully.

"Allie's sister, Bri, didn't have as many problems, but when I first brought her to see you she was always picking her nose, scratching her bottom, grinding her teeth at night, and couldn't wait for anything. You gave her Cina, which cleared up all of those symptoms."

Feedback from a Relieved Teacher

"Luis' transformation after taking his first dose of homeopathic medicine was as immediate as I could have ever imagined. He went from being very unfocused to being an active member of his class. Instead of being aggressive, Luis became aware of, and excited about, learning. He became very involved in classroom projects, especially those with insects, bugs, butterflies, and worms. In fact, he became a real leader. It was a night-and-day kind of change that made all the difference in my work with him. Doors opened for Luis that had been closed to him before. I give homeopathy my raves and raves and raves. I appreciate 100 percent the changes in Luis. I had so much trouble with him before he started homeopathy that I was seriously thinking of quitting my job!"

11

Living with and Learning from a Child with ADHD
Tips for Parents

Here are some suggestions that can help you support your child's healing process.

Appreciate the Uniqueness of Your Child

Recognize how precious your child's special gifts are. Remember—your child is one of a kind (even if there are moments when you wonder if he's the wrong kind!). He may not be what you expected, so let him be himself. One mother of a child with ADHD shared a valuable piece of advice from a physician, which has helped her through many a trying moment with her son. "Imagine," he counseled, "that you are preparing for a wonderful trip to Italy. You get out your map and plan your journey to Florence, Siena, and Rome. Then you take a few classes in Italian. Your mouth is watering at the mere thought of fresh, homemade ravioli. You pack your bags, get on the plane, and you're off to Italia. The plane lands. You look around, bewildered, and realize that you are in Amsterdam, not Italy. Initially you are very disappointed. Then you think about the tulips and the Rembrandts and the windmills and begin to enjoy yourself.

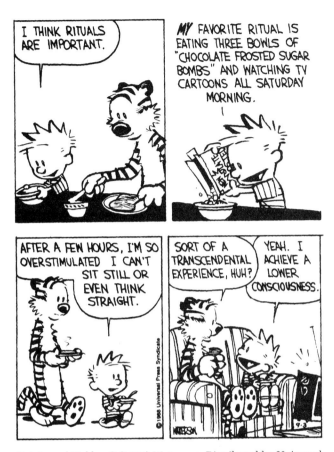

Calvin and Hobbes © (1988) Watterson. Distributed by Universal Press Syndicate. Reprinted with permission. All rights reserved.

You realize that the country is very different. It's not what you expected, but it's still a wonderful place." That's just how it can be with your ADHD child.

Catch Your Kid Doing Something Good

Kids with ADHD usually mean well. They are not trying to be obnoxious, terminally restless, and unbearable to be around. They want to be accepted and liked, to learn and fit in. But the more their behaviors alienate them from their family, teachers, and peers, the worse they feel about themselves. Their self-esteem plummets, whether or not others around them realize it. Most children with ADHD already know they are screwing up. Reminding them of their every mistake only makes them feel more terrible about what they often cannot consciously control.

Whenever you can catch your child doing something good, immediately praise him. Children who are perpetually criticized will live up, or rather down, to their parents' poor expectations of them.

One Step at a Time and Keep It Simple

Children with ADHD have problems following directions, particularly if they are given all at once, in a series. Keep instructions and expectations simple, one at a time. These children may not be known for their ability to multitask, but are often quite capable of completing tasks successfully if they understand just what is expected of them. By asking your child to do one thing at a time, you're increasing the likelihood that he'll succeed. Your child will feel better about his ability to handle demands, and you can positively reinforce each job well done. Once he is capable of simple tasks like brushing his teeth, making his bed, feeding the dog, or taking out the trash, then you can develop more sophisticated strategies, such as chore check-off lists or schedules.

Set Limits and Be Consistent

About 40 percent of kids with ADHD also have tendencies towards defiance. They will bend boundaries to their very limit in an attempt to exert control over their lives. Although an excessively rigid environment can make these kids even more rebellious and defiant, clear, loving limits are essential. Let your child know clearly what you expect and what the consequence will be if she doesn't meet the expectation. Time-outs, restrictions, household chores, and family commitments do not have to be punitive but rather means of establishing firm, reasonable, and consistent guidelines. This is especially important if the parents are divorced, and two households, and sometimes four parents, are involved.

Choose Nonstimulating Activities

Have you ever sat for four hours working on a project or playing computer games? For children who are already overamped, this can be intensely mind-jangling. The same is true of long periods spent in front of the boob tube. Help your child find activities that actually calm her nervous system, such as taking a walk out in nature. Suggest fun activities that burn energy but are not overstimulating, such as swimming, tennis, ice skating, yoga, tai chi, or aikido, as opposed to noisy, fast-paced sports. Many kids with ADHD feel awkward and uncoordinated. Helping them to find a sport or activity in which they can succeed is a great way not only to calm a strung-out nervous system, but also to enhance self-esteem.

Become a Master of Communication with Your Child

Learn what it takes to communicate well with your child. A major problem with ADHD children is that they selectively tune out, taking in part or none of what is said to them. Even if they hear every single word, they often do not acknowledge having taken in the information, and you may feel unheard. Developing successful communication strategies will not only greatly enhance enjoyable conversation with your child, but also provide a model of how she can communicate well with other children. This is particularly important for the type of child with ADHD who feels self-conscious about her inability to express, clams up around other children, and ends up feeling isolated.

Cultivate Your Sense of Humor

Having an ADHD child can push your buttons, make you want to scream, and drive you crazy, but these children can also be hilarious. We are not suggesting that you roll over laughing when your little angel puts your watch in the microwave or pours cement down your kitchen sink. It is not helpful to positively reinforce destructive tendencies, but when appropriate, let yourself become a child again, innocent and spontaneous. No matter how much your child's behaviors upset you, remember to find ways to laugh and have fun together. ADHD children's lives can be filled with many moments of hyperintensity. They need opportunities to lighten up as much as you do.

Don't Let the ADHD Destroy Your Happiness, Sanity, and Marriage

Watch for the red flags that indicate that you are depressed, stuffing rage, or have sunk into a state of apathy about your family and your life. Loving and raising an ADHD child has its many challenges, but do not forget about the rest of your life. This may mean seeking out babysitters or after-school or weekend activities for your child so that you can sometimes get a break. As a parent, you need to cultivate your own peace, happiness, and creativity. It is a big mistake to sublimate your own needs for ten to twenty years while you devote every waking hour to your hyperactive child. Don't lose yourself in the process of raising your family. If the tension generated by your child's behavioral problems creates significant dissention between you and your spouse, partner, or the other children, seek out help in the form of counseling or a support group.

Fight Only the Big Battles

Set clear limits and identify the issues that matter the most. Save your energy for what really matters. Richard Carlson has it right; it really isn't worth it to sweat the small stuff![14] You may want your daughter to bathe every morning, brush her teeth twice a day, and wear clean, ironed clothes to school. She may not care, and the cleanliness issue may develop into an ongoing battle. You may be an ardent vegetarian who feels incensed upon seeing your child scarf down a cheeseburger with fries. You may find chilling out the best solution to save your sanity.

Fighting over every little thing will make your life, as well as your child's life, miserable. It's just not worth it. Compromise. Be clear about those issues on which

[14] Richard Carlson, *Don't Sweat the Small Stuff . . . and It's All Small Stuff* (New York: Hyperion, 1997).

you stand absolutely firm, but give your kid some slack in other areas. Remember the story about Italy and Holland. Admire the tulips even though you were hoping for a romantic dinner of ravioli and Chianti.

Get Treatment for Your Own ADHD

We have found that many children with ADHD have parents with ADHD. The traits may have been merely a mild annoyance in school and no longer interfere with daily life. In other cases, however, the parent has such strong tendencies toward distractibility, hurriedness, forgetfulness, and inability to keep commitments and to follow through on tasks that the child cannot help but be affected. We treated one woman with two children diagnosed with ADHD. She could not remember anything that she had to do unless she wrote it down on two calendars. She even forgot to pick her kids up at school. Other parents could not remember their children's appointments with us if their lives depended on it. If you suffer from ADHD yourself, get help. You will be helping yourself and your family immensely.

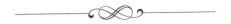

PART THREE

Real Stories of Real People: Successful Homeopathic Treatment of ADHD

12

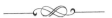

Kids on the Move
Attention Deficit with Hyperactivity

A Teenager on the Go Go Go

Sixteen-year-old Sherrie was referred to us by her family-practice physician because of a five-year history of ADHD. An aunt and a cousin on both sides of the family had also been diagnosed as hyperactive. Her father and maternal aunt suffered from bipolar disorder (manic depression). As early as kindergarten, Sherrie was sent out of the classroom for talking too much. By the sixth grade she was taking Ritalin. Without her Ritalin, Sherrie simply could not focus. Easily distracted by noise or movement, Sherrie found it extremely challenging to pay attention during conversations or to concentrate while taking tests. Sherrie talked without listening and often found herself staring off into space mid-sentence. No matter how much she told herself to be quiet, she could not help but blurt whatever was on her mind, appropriate or not. Sometimes she felt embarrassed, though often she had little, if any, awareness regarding how she affected others. She had a reputation among her friends of being loud, immature, and the last one to catch on to a joke. While driving, she often daydreamed and became confused upon seeing a car in another lane, as if she did not believe it was actually happening.

Antsy, fidgety, and prone to fiddling with anything within her reach, Sherrie perpetually clicked her nails against her teeth, tapped her fingers, poked, hugged, and pulled at others annoyingly. She was simply incapable of keeping her hands to herself. She was always moving some part of her body and skipped down the hall to release her pent-up energy. When there was no way to let it out, she felt like screaming. "The energy is trapped inside of me and has to be pushed out. It's all out of control," she explained.

Ritalin gave Sherrie hives and made her feel like she did not know herself. Nor did it improve her habit of being "a major procrastinator." With or without medication, Sherrie asked lots of "dumb questions," although she maintained a 3.8 grade-point average.

This young woman had a passion for pickles and ate them straight from the jar. She also enjoyed sucking on ice. Her fingers and toes became extremely cold when she skied.

Sherrie's defining features were her extreme restlessness and ceaseless activity. We gave her *Veratrum*

Veratrum album (white hellebore)

Kids who need this medicine are bright even precocious, and restless to the point of being ceaselessly busy. *Veratrum* children touch everything in sight and are always moving on to their next challenge. They think they know it all and can be quite bossy, self-righteous, and given to debate. Some of these children hug and kiss inappropriately. Often chilly, they may have very cold hands and feet, which turn white or blue. Vomiting, diarrhea, and fainting are typical physical symptoms. They love cold food and drinks, ice, pickles, and fruit.

album (white hellebore), an excellent medicine for wired, overamped, hurried kids who are on the move nonstop. These people are generally good-natured and helpful, but overexuberant. Their energy oozes out around the edges. As we frequently do in treating children and adolescents, we gave here a single dose of the medicine and asked her to return in five weeks.

At the time of her next appointment, Sherrie was very happy with her progress, as were her parents. She had informed her psychiatrist that she wanted to discontinue the Ritalin before taking the homeopathic medicine. When she came for her follow-up visit, Sherrie found our parking lot without directions, a task she could normally accomplish only with the help of Ritalin. Her grades were better, in contrast to her previous efforts to discontinue Ritalin, when her grades plummeted to all F's.

Sherrie's parents also reported that her behavior had drastically improved. No longer did she stare blankly. Sherrie's friends complimented her by saying that she "wasn't as crazy" as before. Overall, she felt a much greater sense of control. She was no longer seized with the urge to poke, hug, and pull at other people. Sherrie's leg no longer moved restlessly, nor was she clicking her nails against her teeth. She remarked that she was not as depressed as she had been, although she had not actually described herself that way previously.

Sherrie now had "a real appetite" instead of sporadic urges to eat. She no longer experienced "that special taste for pickles." Sherrie needed two doses of the *Veratrum* over the next year and a half, then discontinued treatment because she felt fine. She did not resume taking Ritalin. As her treatment progressed, Sherrie was able to notice whenever she felt even a little hyperactive and could stop it by telling herself to relax. Before beginning homeopathic treatment, She had been unable to notice or control her behavior patterns. Now she became fidgety only occasionally instead of all the time. When her voice became loud, she quieted down, which had also been impossible in the past. "It's like somebody opened the curtains and let me see."

The Didgeridoo Kid from Down Under

Angela's mother brought her to see us when she was twenty-two months old. The Australian family was visiting the United States during Angela's father's didgeridoo concert tour. The didgeridoo is a rhythmic Aboriginal instrument. Angela had a red rash on her face. She had not gotten one good night's sleep (nor had her parents!) since birth. When her mother weaned her at seven months, Angela refused cow's milk. Angela had a pattern of waking in the middle of the night crying, distressed, and disoriented. Her parents tried to soothe her despair by letting her sleep with them; otherwise she woke repeatedly crying for her mother. This hyper-energetic toddler fought for hours against going to sleep. Her mother described her as being "in a frenzy every night." Angela's exhausted parents had even resorted unsuccessfully to giving their little darling sleeping pills.

Angela was extremely willful. It was very nerve-wracking to travel with her, which conflicted with her father's career as a traveling entertainer. Angela screamed inconsolably at the top of her lungs during most of our interview with her. Even when her mother offered her a bottle of her favorite juice, she refused and threw herself miserably on the floor.

Angela loved people. A lively baby who resisted naps, she lived in an equally vibrant household where friends and family members were constantly coming and going. Angela walked at nine months and ran at ten. An avid climber, she scaled anything within her reach with absolutely no hint of trepidation. She loved playing with animals and putting on her mother's lipstick. When we inquired about this little girl's musical affinity, her mother told us that as soon as the music came on, Angela squirmed and danced. Even at her very young age, she sat at the piano bench and banged on the keys and was thrilled to play her father's guitar while he rocked her on his knee. Family friends were amazed at Angela's rhythmical talents.

Angela had been diagnosed with an unusual skin condition called dermatomyositis, which showed up as purplish, red, scarred areas on her fingers resembling tiny splinters.

We gave Angela one dose of homeopathic *Tarentula*. This medicine, made from the Spanish spider, is for overactive children who are extremely lively, love to be the center of attention, climb like little spiders, and love dancing and rhythmic music. They throw tantrums and fits and can be quite mischievous and manipulative. It is understandable that Angela, raised in an environment of music and dance, needed this lively medicine. A well-respected Italian homeopathic physician, Massimo Mangialavori, recounts a story of a small southern village in Italy near the seaport of Tarent. A group of girls in the village suffered from a hysterical type of insanity that was only relieved when they danced in a type of frenzy and cut with knives or swords.[1] Although it did not come up in Angela's case,

---

[1] M. Pelt, "Spiders in Nature and Homeopathy: Mangialavore in Wageningen, Autumn 1993 and 1994," *Homeopathic Links* 8(3): 45–46 (1995).

many children needing *Tarentula* do have an urge to wildly cut clothing and other things during their rages.

Angela's mother called from Australia five weeks after she took the medicine. Angela had no further tantrums or extreme moodiness; "just the odd two-year-old stuff." Her mother had no complaints about Angela's behavior compared to before she took the *Tarentula*. Now she was much more easily managed when she became upset. She jumped up and down occasionally when her mother said no, but would settle down. Angela was much more easily entertained. It was much easier for her to sit in a car, which had been a major problem previously. Her teeth grinding, which her mother forgot to mention in the first interview, was 90 percent improved. The redness and scarring on her hands were also better. Angela's mother added that prior to the homeopathic treatment, her daughter was forever tapping, teasing, and getting into mischief. These behaviors had also improved. "Looks like Miss Spider's working," her mother exclaimed.

Angela needed one more dose of the *Tarentula* five months later because some of her symptoms had returned, though at a much lower level than before the homeopathic treatment. Angela's dermatologist was quite surprised that the redness and inflammation of her fingers had improved significantly.

I've Been Very Bad!

Conner, age six, was extraordinarily bright. This precocious child started reading at three and was adept at math and language, as well as being highly creative and intuitive. However, his social and interpersonal skills needed work. Quick to anger, he was generally oblivious

Tarentula hispanica (tarantula spider)

Tarentula children have rhythm. These kids love to be the center of attention and can be real entertainers. They climb, jump, perform acrobatics, and seemingly never tire of activity. They love music and rhythmic activities like dancing, tapping, or drumming, and it soothes them. Cunning and mischievous, they play tricks on their parents and other children, tell lies, and love to hide. They are very hurried and impatient. Often destructive, they have to be watched very closely, as they are capable of breaking anything they get their hands on. They are generally wiry and agile.

to social cues. Impulsive, he had taken it upon himself to go through the other children's lunch boxes to see what might appeal to him, then tried to do it again just after being reprimanded. Important lessons were rapidly forgotten.

Hypersensitive to being touched, Conner nonetheless was prone to hugging, tapping, and annoying kids around him. A strong-willed, rather self-righteous child, Conner could be pushing and controlling. Order and morality were so important to Conner that he became quite upset if the other children didn't act in a way that he believed supported these values. When a group of boys were disruptive in class, Conner took the side of his teacher, shouting, "They're not following the rules!"

Conner's teacher considered him to be very hyperactive, and the school psychologist concurred with the diagnosis of ADHD, but Adderall hadn't helped him much, so they took him off of it. Conner's unusual aptitude for arguing led his parents to joke that he would make a great politician or lawyer.

The most unusual feature of Conner was how hard he was on himself. Once, when his parents gave him a time-out, he became semihysterical. Conner claimed he'd done so many bad things in his six years of life that his spirit was going to be wiped off the face of the earth. In fact, he told his parents that it was hard to accept their love because of the terrible things he had done. He magnified the least criticism one hundred-fold.

The recurrent theme in Conner's play was being a lost little boy whose mommy and daddy were dead. He would ask those who passed by, "Will you take me home with you?" Conner had lost his grandfather several years earlier and still felt a strong emotional attachment to him. He still carried on frequent conversations with him. Conner had one recurrent dream in which he was in the middle of a circle of all of his loved ones.

When Conner's mom was seven months pregnant, she and her husband were evicted from their home because it was sold. Insistent that they find a home of their own, they bought a house immediately.

We thought it odd that Conner should be so tormented by guilt as well as having the recurrent fear of being orphaned. It turned out that his mother had forged several checks ten years before Conner's birth, for which she spent one year in jail. "I went through hell as a result of being caught and convicted," she confided. We, and other homeopaths, observe on a regular basis that the thoughts and feelings that the parents experience immediately prior to conception or during the pregnancy can have a direct effect of the state of the child. The younger the child, the clearer is this hereditary influence, regardless of whether it is passed on genetically or by some other mechanism. As a child grows, it may be harder to separate out nature versus nurture (what is inherited compared with what a child learns from his environment).

With this additional information, we were quite sure of Conner's prescription and inquired whether he had any tendency to restless or busy hands. His parents confirmed that he was prone to making frequent inappropriate hand and body motions, as well as reaching out to touch people, even strangers. We gave Conner *Kali bromatum* (potassium bromate), an excellent medicine for upright, family-oriented individuals who feel as if they have sinned away their day of grace and must be punished by God. Conner had clearly inherited this feeling state from his mother due to her criminal behavior a number of years prior to conception.

At our six-week appointment, Conner was behaving much better in social situations. His need to touch was reduced, as was as his compulsive need for order. When we spoke a couple of months later, his mom reported that Conner was much more pleasant, reasonable, less fidgety, and more forgiving of himself. Now, three years after beginning homeopathic treatment, Conner is still doing well. He has needed three doses of the medicine each year. The feedback from the school is that he is much more attentive in class, willing to try new things more than ever before, has a more positive outlook, and was able to have fun with the other children at recess. Conner's parents are very happy with his progress.

A Sweet, Squirmy Kid

Michael was diagnosed with ADHD at age six. His pediatrician prescribed Ritalin, but his mother was not comfortable with medicating her son. Michael's teachers complained about his squirminess, pouting, sulking; worrying, inappropriate noises; immature behavior; and distractibility, restlessness, and disruptiveness. Next on the list of unacceptable behaviors were excitability, impulsivity, sucking, chewing, frequent crying, tendency to become easily frustrated, boasting, hypersensitivity to criticism, daydreaming, excessive demands for teacher's attention, submissiveness, and failure to complete tasks. How's that for a list!

Test scores made it appear that Michael had significant learning and behavior problems, but the child we saw in our office was sweet and sensitive. His mother described him as "pretty darn average—like any other six-year-old kid, but more active." Michael definitely had difficulty sitting still in school. His work was inconsistent. "Some of his papers were done perfectly, others looked like an alien completed them." Michael preferred to socialize rather than do his homework. Teachers noticed that his behavior was fantastic one day and terrible the next.

Michael became wound up very easily, especially when bored. He entertained himself by crumpling up little scraps of paper and throwing them away one at a time. Michael needed to be in constant motion, sometimes ran out of the classroom eight to ten times a day to go to the bathroom, or crawled around on the floor in class. To make matters worse, he would not stop after the teacher reprimanded him the first time.

Focusing at home was no easier for Michael. If the television was on or the curtains open, his mom had to make him repeat back what she told him or he would not respond. Michael was never violent or aggressive and tended to be a follower. Kids loved him because they thought he was funny, but his self-confidence was really low.

Michael's parents divorced when he was two years old. He was never sure when his dad would come pick him up. A pleaser, he worried about his father's violence toward his stepmother, about being late for school, about his shoelaces breaking, and about having enough money for lunch. He was also preoccupied with who would pick him up from school and how many days he would stay with his dad.

An overly sensitive child, Michael cried if reprimanded even gently. "It scares me when somebody yells at me. I'm afraid I'll have to be on restriction again. I get really upset at myself." Michael really wanted to be good and felt awful about himself when he messed up and got into trouble.

We found many apparent contradictions in Michael. Disruptive and inappropriate, he was highly sensitive. Michael was alternately sulky and loving. Fearful of making mistakes, he acted out anyway. Many of his symptoms were classic ADHD symptoms that did not differentiate him from the many other children diagnosed with ADHD—impulsivity, excitability,

Natrum muriaticum (sodium chloride)

The main feeling in children needing *Natrum muriaticum,* derived from table salt, is feeling rejected and unloved, and then withdrawing to avoid being hurt again. These children tend to be shy, introverted, and rarely present behavior problems. They cry their salty tears alone, not wanting to be embarrassed in public. They tend to be confidantes to parents or to friends. Headaches, allergies, and cold sores are common complaints. The kids often crave salt, pasta, and bread, and are averse to slimy foods and fat.

distractibility, and difficulty maintaining focus. Yet, unlike many children with ADHD, he felt very guilty about his unacceptable behaviors and constantly worried about "messing up." Most children who are naughty are not overly sensitive pleasers. It was this combination of typical ADHD symptoms and oversensitive and excessive worrying that stood out about Michael in our eyes.

Michael responded extremely well to one dose of *Natrum muriaticum* (sodium chloride)—a medicine given to very sensitive people, often after grief or loss. People needing this medicine are unusually sensitive to reprimands and tend to feel very bad about themselves when they do something wrong. Michael has needed this medicine only two times over the past year. Within weeks of beginning treatment, Michael's teachers were amazed at the tremendous improvement in his attitude and behavior. His continual movement had diminished. Before homeopathic treatment, Michael received four to five checks (corresponding to reprimands) a day. By his follow-up visit six weeks after starting homeopathy, he had not received even one check. Michael was no longer so sensitive to reprimands.

When we asked Michael how he felt, he replied, "It's easier to concentrate. Sometimes I'm getting stars and superstars and Mommy's really proud of me." What was most touching about seeing the changes in Michael was how much better he felt about himself.

Michael's improvement has continued. He no longer acts out in class or at lunch. He stays in his seat more and does not worry as much. His leadership skills have improved tremendously. He was recently chosen "student of the week." The biggest improvement the teacher has noticed is his effort. Everyone is just thrilled with Michael's behavior.

13

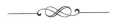

"I Have to Tell Him Everything Ten Times"
Attention Deficit Without Hyperactivity

Some parents ask us, "Are all of your cases extreme? My child just has a mild case of ADHD." Let us assure you that, although some of the children in our books may be climbing the walls, punching out their classmates, or behaving in an impossibly impulsive way, many of the kids we see are your garden-variety, otherwise normal, nice children who just can't concentrate. Such are the children in this chapter.

He Cannot Hang On to Directions

Grace brought in her son Jeff when he was eight. Under evaluation for ADHD at the local children's hospital, he was unable to sit still and pay attention in the classroom. Kindergarten had been a nightmare for Jeff. His attitude was terrible, staying in his seat was impossible, and he jumped up every few minutes to sharpen pencils or chatter with friends. Anything and everything distracted Jeff. His mind drifted constantly. His mother explained, "He can even hear the grass grow." Jeff simply could not hang on to a direction if his life depended on it. Mouthy in class, he led his teachers to lose patience with him quickly because of his incessant interruptions and disruption. This youngster conveniently forgot to tell his mother when he got into trouble at school. Jeff had serious academic problems. Held back in the first grade due to his inability to read, by the beginning of second grade, when his mother first consulted us, Jeff was writing his numbers and letters backward.

Jeff's parents divorced when he was three, which affected him deeply. His behavior regressed for several years afterwards and he refused to stop nursing. He was very insecure, "a momma's boy," and became frightened easily. Jeff was charming and sweet with adults and younger children, but shy with kids his own age and had difficulty making friends. Jeff seemed starved for attention and insisted, "Watch me, watch me!"

Jeff experienced enormous mood swings and was described by his mother as "happy as a lark or mad as a hornet." He cried, screamed, swore, slammed doors, and alternately told his mother that he loved and hated her. When angry, Jeff became wild, throwing things on the floor and ripping up paper.

Life was scary for Jeff. Afraid to look out of the windows at night, he slept in bed with his brother until recently because he was afraid to be alone. He feared the dark and slept with a night-light. Jeff held his mother's hand while watching scary movies until he was seven years old. Jeff didn't want to try anything new, particularly if he wasn't sure he would succeed at it the first time.

Jeff's physical complaints included diarrhea, stomachaches, and a constant runny nose. He loved chicken, sweets, and hamburgers. Jeff became wound up and wild after eating sugar.

The medicine that benefited Jeff the most was *Lycopodium* (club moss). It can help fearful children who act immaturely and try to cover up their mistakes. They make every effort to appear courageous and powerful, but inside they are timid and afraid. Kids like Jeff often feel more comfortable playing with younger children rather than their peers, because they feel older and can boss the younger children around. These children are very concerned with what others think and try to look cool at all costs. A deep insecurity inside often causes them to feel very anxious about performing in public or taking examinations. They fear that their inner weakness or lack of mastery might be revealed. There may also be a tendency to dyslexia and distractibility. These children often could die for sweets but can also have bad reactions, physically or behaviorally.

Lycopodium clavatum (club moss)

Those needing this medicine are often fearful and cowardly but try not to show it. Inside they feel inadequate and lack self-confidence, often having been raised by parents who constantly put them down and tell them they cannot do anything right. These children boss others around, especially children younger than themselves, and may even assume the role of the class clown. They can be distractible and dyslexic. People needing *Lycopodium* are reluctant to try new things because they fear they will fail. The most prominent food craving is sweets, and there is a tendency toward hypoglycemia. Physical symptoms often include gas and bloating, particularly from beans and the cabbage family.

Two months after he was given the medicine, Jeff got his highest marks ever in school. His dyslexia was improving. He was able to sit still, raise his hand, and pay attention in class. Over the next eighteen months, Jeff's behavior steadily improved. Able to make new friends more easily, the other kids began to look up to Jeff because he was so agile in sports. Less impulsive, Jeff was reported by his teachers to have improved dramatically in his behavior. He accomplished two years of math in six months. For the first time, the teachers recognized that Jeff was very bright. They removed him from special-education classes where his unruly behavior had landed him. Now, three years after beginning homeopathy, he continues to do very well in a mainstream classroom.

A Spaced Out Kid

Twelve-year-old Colin's mom called us first two years ago seeking help for her son's difficulty with paying attention. His dad estimated that instructions that he gave to Colin didn't register 70 to 80 percent of the time. "We first began to notice a problem with focus and learning during the third grade. At first we thought it was personality conflict with his teacher, so we dismissed it. But, by the fourth, all of his teachers observed that he was struggling to keep up. They agreed that he didn't seem to attend to instructions, so they had to repeat them for Colin. Or, if did comprehend the directions, he couldn't finish the material in time, or he would turn in papers late. All of his teachers have told us since then that Colin seems like he's out in space and they have to call back to get him to focus. It's awfully hard to get him to finish his homework. He gets antsy and has to get up

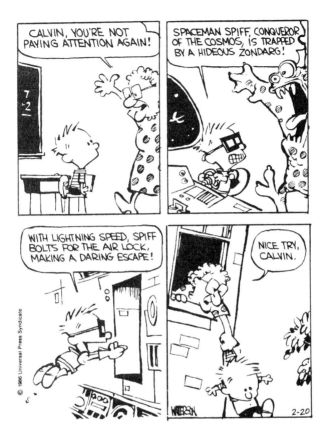

Calvin and Hobbes © (1986) Watterson. Distributed by Universal Press Syndicate. Reprinted with permission. All rights reserved.

and walk around or he might not even remember what he's supposed to do. He reads well, and he's not bad at math. If he's doing something he really, really likes, like Nintendo, Colin stays right on it, but if the task is boring or monotonous, he simply can't stay on track. They've diagnosed him with mild ADHD. We gave him Ritalin for two months in the fourth grade, but I didn't want to continue giving him drugs.

"Colin just drifts, daydreams, stares off into the distance. 'Spaced out' is what everyone says about him.

The teachers call us frequently to complain about his inattentiveness. His dreaminess has definitely hurt his grades, although he's never failed at anything. He's just at a lower level. He used to be in the highest level reading group, but not anymore. Colin talks, giggles, whistles, acts silly, and talks during class and is put in detention for disrupting his classmates. Then he has to ask his teacher what he is supposed to be doing."

"Colin will get some idea in his head about what he wants to do, and he won't let go of it, even though knows he'll get into trouble. I told him he couldn't watch wrestling on television because he hadn't finished his homework. I gave him three or four warnings, but he didn't listen. The consequence was not going to a movie that he really wanted to see."

Colin was energy-packed, and it was hard to get him to settle down at night, especially during the school year, then it was even more challenging to get him up in the morning. A dawdler, it was a huge struggle to get him moving and ready for school. In the past, Colin was a sweet child who longed to please, but lately he had become sassy with his mom. Generally not a big talker, Colin tended to mumble and could seem unfriendly if he was not in the mood to talk, but friends were not a problem for him. Colin was a kind-hearted kid who cared about people. He talked more freely with his dad than his mom, and she felt baffled by how the Colin that she knew could get into so much trouble at school.

"One of his best friends was accidentally shot to death last year. It really hit Colin hard. He cried just about every night for four or five months. He was so considerate to the other people who were affected by it. He seems to be changing, though. Acts up in church with his friends and he's a bit reckless lately, especially with his go-kart. Colin gets up and doesn't even let me know where he's going. He just walks off. The other day he took off on his go-kart and had a pretty bad wreck. A man who saw it told me afterward that Colin was going way too fast and he just flew right off of it. He could have gotten badly hurt. He's even been known to play with matches a few times." Colin's mother mentioned that it was difficult to think clearly herself.

We inquired about any past history of head injuries. That jogged his mom's memory to recall a time when he was in the second grade, playing outside with his sister on a pulley, swinging from one tree to another. Before he knew it, the pulley hit him right smack in the forehead. His teacher reported that Colin fell forward on his desk the following day. A neurological examination and electroencephalogram were normal.

When we asked Colin about his concentration, he replied, "No problem. It's just that I don't pay attention sometimes or I talk to people." The degree of awareness and insight that kids have about themselves varies greatly. Colin, though kind and well meaning, seemed as tuned out about himself as he did about the world around him.

The first medicine that we prescribed for Colin, *Calcarea carbonica,* produced a partial improvement in many of his symptoms. Six months after we first saw Colin, he was again "drifting, daydreamy, and out in space—as if he were in another world." A repetition of the *Calcarea carbonica* unfortunately no longer helped, so we changed Colin's medicine to *Helleborus* (black hellebore). This is an excellent medicine for tuned-out, drifty kids who can be oblivious to the world around them. It is also indicated for the after-effects of head injuries and grief.

Seven weeks later Colin's mom was happy to report a dramatic improvement. Colin's grades were up, and his attention was so much improved that he had made the honor roll! More able to control his talking, giggling, and distractedness, he was also performing well in sports. What made his mom the happiest was that Colin had finally joined the planet. The rash on his arms that had bothered him was gone, and his athlete's foot was considerably better.

Three months later Colin's name continued to grace the honor roll, his teachers were very pleased, and his mother was proud to say that he was much more out-going. Attentive at home and at school, able to converse normally in a variety of settings, he had, according to his mom, improved an estimated 80 percent since starting homeopathic treatment. This positive change has continued to the extent that we now have appointments with Colin only every six months.

"I Won't Grow Up!"

"We have no idea who Melissa's father is," her adoptive mother began. "We adopted her at birth." Melissa's birth mom got pregnant at eighteen, dropped out of high school, "did a lot of crazy things," and was a pathological liar. Her mother described the seven-year-old little girl as "sweet, but an airhead." The maternal grandmother would have nothing to do with her daughter or the baby. The birth mom was not sure of the father's identity. If he were the man she suspected, he was also pretty crazy and quite the risk-taker. Neither of them thought much about consequences. Soon after Melissa's birth, the mother became pregnant again and asked that the adoptive family take that child too. They declined, but did find another family to adopt the sibling.

A good baby, Melissa hardly cried, yet experienced night terrors from the age of one week. She was never interested in eating, and her adoptive mom still had to force her to eat. All of the other children thought she was a riot because she sang and danced her way up to front of class, but Melissa just couldn't focus. The first grade teacher reported that she chatted with her neighbors, stared out the window, dilly dallied, and was forever being sidetracked. "She just doesn't think," her mom explained. At least eight months behind her peers in maturity, Melissa fell into frequent crying jags. During these episodes, she insisted that she only wanted to play and would never grow up. Melissa's favorite playmates were several years younger than herself. At first she refused to be around, and even appeared to dislike, babies. Now she loved spending time with them.

This child's favorite and frequent pastime was imitating animals. In kindergarten, she pretended to be a dog to the point of trying her teacher's patience or strutted around like a kitty cat. Melissa adored the family Bishon and surrounded herself with "zillions of stuffed animals," especially little ones like Beanie Babies™. When younger, Melissa stuck out her tongue and pretended to lick like a dog. Now, her parting words to her grandmother on leaving for school each morning were, "Aarf, aarf." Melissa's attraction to animals was so strong that her mom even enrolled her in a monthly experiential program at the local zoo. Melissa even told me about her recurrent dream of being chased by an alligator. The only kind of animal Melissa was not attracted to was insects. Quite the opposite. Terror-stricken when a moth flew into the car, she also thought it like the end of the world if a fly came into her vicinity. She hated anything flying around her, even a butterfly.

A remarkably persistent child and incessant talker (even more so after eating sweets), Melissa did not let up until she got what she wanted. If she didn't, she would regress to a babyish behavior such as screaming, crying, and pouting. When reprimanded, Melissa lamented to her mom, "You don't love me." An affectionate child "without a mean bone in her body," Melissa loved and sought to be friends with everyone she met and was quick to embrace them in a bear hug. The family had recently moved to another state and a new school, which made Melissa feel even more left out. She frequently complained, "Nobody will play with me!" Melissa insisted on being around other kids as much as possible, but, when she was, she was right in their faces, which made them avoid her. She so missed her best friend who had moved to Chicago that her mom arranged a phone call between the two once a week. Loneliness also crept in at night, first in the form of night terrors. Later she began crawling into her parents' bed in the middle of the night.

Melissa's very favorite foods were chocolate ice-cream cones and Eskimo Pies, but her mom was hesitant to give them to her because of her grouchiness after eating chocolate. Earlier in her life, chocolate also gave her large, red blotches on the forehead. Red candy, beets, and raw carrots were next on Melissa's preferred foods list.

We chose to give Melissa homeopathic *Chocolate* because of her regression to childish behavior, refusal to grow up, feeling of exclusion, affectionateness, attraction to, imitation of, and dreams about animals, and her strong desire for chocolate and for red foods. Chocolate is excellent medicine for children who feel either that their mothers did not properly nurture them or that they missed out on the playfulness of childhood, resulting in a Peter Pan-like insistence on never growing up.

Melissa's mom reported six weeks later that she was arguing less, was willing to eat foods she had refused previously, no longer engaged in animal-like behavior, and was now taking care of the younger children like a little mother. "She's growing up!" Melissa chattered and interrupted less and was becoming generally more independent. Within three months, her parents reported that her symptoms were 75 to 80 percent improved.

Seven months after our first appointment, Melissa's parents assured us that both they and her teachers were quite pleased with how much more easily she paid attention and finished her schoolwork. The daydreaming had diminished considerably, and the improvement in her ability to do homework was "like night and day." Melissa's mom described the changes in her daughter as "wonderful," "amazing," "a complete turnaround," and was thrilled that her daughter was now "acting like a regular kid." Melissa no longer pretended she was an animal, was now polite and caring with other kids rather than acting "babyish and bratty," and had even made a new friend. The incessant talking now occurred only after eating too much sugar, and her argumentativeness had vanished. Melissa's mom estimated the overall improvement at 95 per cent. She has needed no treatment over the past four months.

"I Hate Math and Spelling! I Can't Do Anything!"

Hope's problem, from the time she was a toddler, was focusing. Never a child who was able to sit down with crayons and entertain herself, Hope would shift continuously from one activity to the next. Her mom described it as being unable to "settle." Raised and educated in Europe, Hope acted much less mature than her peers. The combination of her difficulty sticking with a task and a lazy eye made it impossible for her to complete her reading assignments. Her parents were so concerned that they moved the entire family to the United States where they hoped her attention deficits might be better addressed. Nevertheless, by the end of the second grade, Hope's vocabulary was advanced, but she simply couldn't read. Nor were her math skills at grade level. Memorizing multiplication tables was out of Hope's reach.

When Hope's mother first called us, she was almost done with the fourth grade and, even with the help of a daily private tutor, she could not sustain her attention in the classroom. Hope was in no way a disruptive child. Her teachers found her delightful, but her mind simply wandered.

This little girl was a hard worker who really wanted to succeed, but couldn't. "I just can't do anything," she lamented to her parents. Highly sensitive to criticism, she feared being wrong and her ego became increasingly deflated. "I hate math. I hate spelling. I'm never going to university," Hope insisted. She was hyperaware of where she stood in her class ratings, even down to the last spelling word. Upon reaching her frustration threshold, she shut down completely and refused to read anything at all. Hope's mom described it as "a veil" that prevented learning from entering her little girl's mind.

A charming, affectionate, mischievous, even impish, child, Hope charmed everyone who met her and made them want to be around her. She was just like her mom in this regard, and anyone who saw them together remarked on their striking resemblance, right down to the haircut. Attracting friends and keeping up conversations were no problem. But when she became utterly frustrated, Hope shut the door to her room and tore it apart. Her dissatisfaction with herself led her to be more aggressive. This behavior culminated in her not being invited to the birthday party of a really close friend and snapped her back, which made Hope quite sad.

In stark contrast to her lack of confidence academically, Hope was a talented skier and speed skater, an excellent communicator, and loved to travel. She even wore roller blades to her first appointment with us. A girl with strong willpower, she had bitten her nails all her life, but had recently decided to quit and did just that. Fitting into her peer group and being liked were high on Hope's scale of values. If the crowd were doing something, so would she. This led to impulsivity and questionable judgment. Even if she had done something that was clearly wrong, Hope often stood by her story to avoid blame.

Hope was a much-wanted child. Due to two earlier miscarriages, her mother was instructed by her obstetrician to stay in bed for the entire pregnancy. She followed his instructions and, despite severe morning sickness and one episode of bleeding early in her pregnancy, all went well.

Desirous of lots of physical affection and support, Hope always felt much better when her parents were around. She loved company, hated playing alone, and would rather stay inside and do nothing than go out to play by herself. Quite fearful of new situations, Hope was particularly afraid of doctors who might want to help her to focus better.

Hope was not a girl with lots of problems. Overall upbeat and happy-go-lucky, she was weighed down mainly by her inability to focus, leading to frustration and lack of success. She had a terrible fear of having demands put on her that could not fulfill. Hope's mother feared that, as she headed into adolescence, she would constantly compare herself to her classmates. Hope's only physical complaints were headaches from overstress or overstimulation and knee pain dating back to a skiing injury.

We first gave Hope *Calcarea phosphorica* (calcium phosphate) due to her concentration difficulties, tremendous frustration, athletic nature, friendliness, desire to travel, and a history of an ankle fracture at age seven. We were definitely not satisfied with the slight improvement that resulted. Hope's mother again emphasized that the most pressing problem was her intense frustration around what she considered to be failure.

At the two-month point, we changed Hope's prescription to *Carcinosin* (nosode), an excellent medicine for children (and adults) who aspire to high, even unreasonable, achievements and have a pattern of stretching themselves to and beyond their limits.

It was over three months when we spoke again with her mother. She had wanted to wait until Hope had been in school for a month to get an accurate idea of how she was faring. "I think we're on the right path," she assured us. "She is much more balanced and calm. No more rages. I would call her 'on' rather than 'switched on.'" Her tutor found her much more able to focus and her self-confidence regarding academics was much improved. Hope had progressed steadily in her reading, was less fearful of new situations, and more considerate. Her headaches were gone as well as the knee pain, despite running a five-kilometer race. "Being more balanced sums it all up," explained her mom.

Hope has needed three more doses of *Carcinosin* over the past seven months. In a recent phone consultation, her mother exclaimed that Hope received the best report card in her life, including an A-plus in science and a B in reading, although math was still a challenge. She even received an award for outstanding achievement. "Hope has relief written all over her," commented her mother. "I'd say she was 75 percent better all around."

14

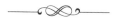

"You Never Know What She's Up To"
Sneaky, Mischievous Kids

Many of us read the comic strip "Dennis the Menace" growing up. Dennis's contemporary counterpart, who mischievously traverses the pages of this book, is Calvin. Sneaky children are at their best engaging, entertaining, and humorous. When carried to its limits, however, mischievousness can drive a parent to desperation. A child may carry teasing and hiding to dangerous extremes. Lying and stealing may follow. What began as good-hearted play can turn into harmful, destructive, or even criminal behavior. All of the children whose cases we share in this chapter are good-natured, but all engage in inappropriate behaviors.

"He Acts First and Thinks Later"

Fourteen-year-old Phil was a likable, engaging young man. His mother's main complaints were that he acted before he thought and was erratic and compulsive. "He does crazy things. He likes to be in the spotlight. He can be in the middle of dribbling in a basketball game, and he'll stop and do a little dance with the ball. He's a very funny kid, like one of the Marx brothers. He cracks me up. He totally dismantled a karate class of fifty kids with his antics. The teacher completely lost control of the class because everyone was doubled over laughing." Phil had a dramatic streak. Despite a stammer, he tended to talk too loudly and be excessively exuberant. He was good at playing piano, but he only enjoyed music with a fast rhythm and pace.

Phil had his tricky side—once he flicked lit matches and threw them on cars. He had a habit of lying compulsively. While his parents slept, he would raid the refrigerator and then deny it later. His hands could be full of ice cream and sticky buns, and still he would play Mr. Innocent. This young man took magazines, baseball cards, and other special possessions from his brother's room without batting an eyelid. Ever a manipulator, Phil had a habit of pushing as far as he could. He did not like to be teased and had a low threshold for adversity. When he lost his temper, he swore, threw things, crashed around, and slammed doors.

He was universally liked and had an excellent sense of humor, but could not make friends easily. According to his mom, "Phil could charm a bird out of a tree." Phil was kind to animals and pets and was infinitely patient with the family dog. He was always the one who asked about his mom when she was sick. He sometimes asked for free toys for his sister.

At the same time, Phil's mom was disgusted by his sloppy habits. He lounged in front of the television snacking. He threw orange peels behind the furniture. His mother was constantly discovering dirty socks, Popsicle sticks, candy wrappers, and various remains of snacks turned science projects. It was hard to get Phil to do anything helpful around the house. If she asked him to fold towels, he would stuff them under a couch cushion. It seemed to be a kind of extreme carelessness.

Phil was homeschooled. He was not great at math or penmanship, but was a whiz at Nintendo. He learned best by teaching himself. He was fascinated by UFOs, ghosts, and the Loch Ness monster. He was very frightened by spiders, especially very big ones, but loved reading about tarantulas.

At six, Phil was put on Ritalin without success. He was now on Cylert. He was already an erratic sleeper, and Cylert often kept him up at night. Phil's excesses might include eating nine oranges in a row. He loved pizza.

You can see that Phil was both a character and a study in contradictions. He was lively yet lazy, kind and caring yet lied and stole, was humorous yet filled with rage. Phil loved to be the center of attention, was charming, and often cagey.

We prescribed *Tarentula* for Phil. In addition to his sneakiness, charming nature, tendency to lie, and desire to entertain and get attention, he even mentioned his fear of and fascination with spiders.

The six-week follow-up indicated positive changes in Phil. His mother had noticed a big change in his attitude. He had discontinued the Cylert, gotten a part-time job, and made a new friend. He was sleeping more and longer. Phil felt calmer, not as angry and jittery. He was lying less and had stopped swearing or throwing things. The stammering was also better, and he no longer talked as loudly. He was not pushing his mother to the limits. When people teased Phil, he did not react as angrily as he used to. His mother described him as more even-keeled. He was still a slob around the house.

Nine weeks later Phil continued to do well. He was still calmer and not as belligerent and had no more angry outbursts. He started volunteering at a local community center to help other kids play ball. He told us that he was now thinking differently about his actions and was not as sensitive when teased. He actually folded some towels instead of wadding them up.

Nine and a half months after the dose of *Tarentula*, we asked Phil's mother to assess his progress since he began homeopathic treatment. "It's a night-and-day difference from last year. He's a nicer guy to be around. He isn't as volatile. He doesn't fly off the handle and isn't as nervous. He now has four or five friends and is able to get along with his peers much better. They seem to genuinely like him. He rolls with the punches. The basketball coach complimented him on his playing."

He Loved to Play Tricks on His Teachers

Dennis was a ten-year-old handful. He was a very active, creative kid. He had a bent for comedy and loved to play tricks on his teachers. He enjoyed "scaring the heck out of little kids." Dennis was defiant, argumentative, and "chafed under rules." He was an expert at bucking authority. He was always getting into trouble at school, so his teacher asked him to keep a behavior diary. Dennis pushed the limits to the max. Living with him was like having to read the fine print on contracts every day. People who interacted with Dennis often felt "taken" by him.

A born ham, Dennis constantly sought attention. He loved to act and dance, and was always inventing new steps. He went to great efforts to stand out in a crowd. He loved mimicry and could talk a mile a minute. Dennis's mother remarked, "If electricity fails, just plug in Dennis." He had energy to burn. He played the cello. Classical music put him to sleep, and rock kept him awake. Dennis also had a precocious interest in girls.

Dennis had a strong fear of heights and a milder fear of being chased by dogs. He had a dream of a little guy with spider arms. In his dream a huge boulder exploded and a spider with a red rear-end sat on top of the boulder.

Dennis had a history of bad ear and sinus infections, allergies, and asthmatic bronchitis. His mother hoped that homeopathy could help Dennis with his susceptibility to allergies as well as his behavioral problems.

You have probably noticed the many similarities between Phil and Dennis. They are both live wires and real charmers with a defiant streak. Perhaps Phil, being four years older, just had a little more time to elaborate his act. We also gave *Tarentula* to Dennis. The mischievous quality often found in those needing this medicine calls forth the image of Dennis the Menace. Notice that both Phil and Dennis liked to dance, which is typical of those needing this medicine.

Dennis became "less manic" after the *Tarentula*. Eight months after beginning homeopathy, Dennis won a citizenship award at school. He even chose to complete extra credit. A couple of months later he was on the safety patrol squad and was volunteering to help younger children. He mentioned being scared of bugs that "come and wrap you in cocoons and suck you dry" like a program he saw on television.

It has now been nineteen months since Dennis began homeopathy, and his behavior has continued to earn glowing reports. He still likes to make funny faces, be a comic, and do whatever he can to attract girls.

Luis Hid in the Bushes and His Babysitter Called the Police

Five-year-old Luis had sparkling eyes and a very mischievous grin, as if he had a big secret. His preschool teacher referred him to us. He was very loving, but could be defiant and disruptive at school. Things set him off for no apparent reason. Luis was impulsive and curious, sometimes to the detriment of himself and others. When he went for class walks in the park, he would run out into the street defiantly. If he did not want to hold the hand of another child, as he was instructed to do, he would throw himself down on the sidewalk and have to be carried back to his preschool. His teacher was at the end of her rope, and he was on the verge of being asked to leave the school.

He loved to wander off and hide. He would disappear and not come when called, and he seemed to get a real rise out of teasing people this way. His mischievousness caused quite a problem for his babysitter one time when she could not find him. The frantic sitter called the police, and Luis popped up moments later from the bushes with a smirk. He also had quite a reputation for stealing sprinklers from the neighbors' yards, which was particularly unpopular during dry spells.

Luis's creativity and imagination were boundless. He wrote pages and pages of inventive stories. He drew a wonderful, intricate picture of a big spider. As he narrated the picture, Luis explained that when the spider died, it would feed the earth. He also loved to draw pictures of caterpillars.

Luis had a hard time sitting still during meals. He would pester his brother, tease, poke, and fidget. If he be-

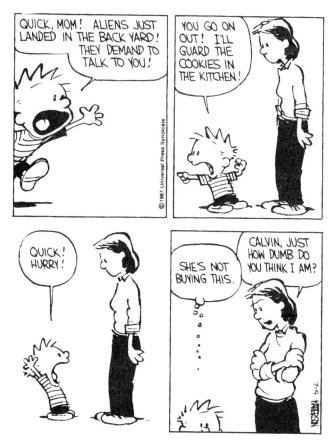

Calvin and Hobbes © (1987) Watterson. Distributed by Universal Press Syndicate. Reprinted with permission. All rights reserved.

came bored at lunch, he would break plastic silverware and toss his food around. He loved to be the leader and tried to get other children to do what he wanted. When he got into a disagreement with his sister, he could hit, kick, and pinch. It was often hard to discipline Luis because he cleverly sidestepped the consequences of his misdeeds with a hug or a kiss. He could also be sneaky about taking things from his brother's room and hiding them while pretending he knew nothing at all about it. When he was younger, he cut his clothes and hair and blamed someone else. He invented an elaborate story about a cat that cut his shorts.

Luis was afraid of monsters coming out of his closet and of shadows on the walls. During storms he would turn on all of the table lamps in his room. He was so sensitive to noises, such as vacuum cleaners, lawn mowers, and chain saws, that he sometimes wore earmuffs to dampen the sound. He was very loving with animals, except for spiders and bugs, which he liked to kill.

Luis was very cute and just a bit too much of a tease for his own good. He was bright, clever, and almost too curious. His special attraction to spiders and bugs interested us. What was most striking about Luis was his desire to hide from other people, no matter what the consequences. Luis had the characteristic restlessness and desire to be the center of attention of *Tarentula,* but no particular love of lively music and dance. We chose for Luis another homeopathic medicine made from a spider, *Aranea ixobola,* a medicine that is specific for people who tease others excessively.

Luis's parents were new to homeopathy and did not know quite what to expect. They were increasingly pleased with the results. The improvement in Luis's attitude began one week after he started homeopathic treatment. The preschool teachers reported that he was more focused and noticeably less defiant, distractible, and disruptive. His mother found him to be happier and less angry. Instead of staying up late at night, he went to sleep more easily. The hiding stopped. Luis listened better. He did not hop up from the table as often during meals, and stuck with tasks longer. He had not hit, kicked, or thrown himself on the floor. During the follow-up interview, Luis talked about digging up worms.

Progress continued beautifully with Luis. He briefly needed a different homeopathic medicine, *Histaminum,* for his allergies. His spirit of exploration blossomed. With his father's help, he slid down the laundry chute at home. The only time he would lose control was when he was terribly hungry or tired. For the past three years, Luis has not needed further treatment.

15

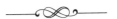

"If I Say Black, He Says White"
Oppositional, Defiant Behavior

All children have stubborn moments. Some have stubborn years. The youngsters in this chapter are more than strong-willed, let-me-do-it kids. They are downright defiant. They can outsmart adults' most skillful distraction techniques and drive their parents crazy by matter-of-factly digging their heels into the ground. No matter is too small to argue about for a determinedly oppositional kid. A sibling suggests one restaurant, the oppositional child insists on another. Burgers were his favorite food until you made them for dinner. Even the simplest of tasks or events like getting dressed for school or eating dinner can become major battlegrounds. Kids like these wear their parents to a frazzle.

Encompassed in the diagnostic category of Oppositional-Defiant Disorder are whining, breath holding, tantrums; arguing with adults; actively defying or refusing requests or rules; deliberately annoying others; blaming others for his every mistake; touchy or easily annoyed by others; angry and resentful; spiteful or vindictive; and swearing.[2] Approximately 40 percent of kids

[2] Carolyn S. Schroeder and Betty N. Gordon, *Assessment and Treatment of Childhood Problems* (New York: The Guilford Press, 1991), 273.

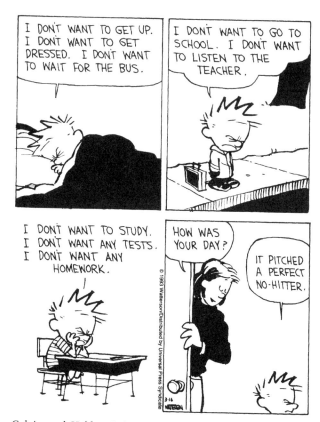

Calvin and Hobbes © (1993) Watterson. Distributed by Universal Press Syndicate. Reprinted with permission. All rights reserved.

with ADHD are also diagnosed with oppositional-defiant disorder, and many display aggression, though we wait until the next chapter to focus on violent behavior.

"I Try to Be Good But My Head Doesn't Let Me"

Darin, age five, had been diagnosed with ADHD one month before his parents called us. They had opted to try

Ritalin first. The medication did improve his concentration, but his mother preferred a more natural alternative.

Darin smiled as the interview began. His mother explained that he had difficulty following instructions. Darin's mother homeschooled him, but she couldn't seem to find a teaching approach that worked for him. Both mother and son became frustrated on a regular basis. When she told us that he had started daycare at three, Darin corrected her. "No, I was two." He did not have a good time playing by himself. He needed a lot of reassurance that he was being good or doing the right thing. He frequently asked his mother, "Am I being good?" or "Am I being quiet?" Darin often told his mother, "I try to be good, to do the right thing, but my head doesn't let me."

Darin had problems listening and following rules. His mother had to ask him again and again to do things. He just didn't seem to act on her requests. Specific problem areas were being unable to settle down at night to go to sleep, to stay quiet, and to stop bothering his brother. "Darin gets really unhappy when he's reprimanded. It makes him cry. He just wants to be good. It takes time for him to settle down at night. I have to go in three times and eventually spank him five nights out of seven to get him to go to sleep. The wrestling, kicking, and hitting are hard to stop.

"The feedback from preschool is that he has difficulty settling down for structured activities. He is unable to sit still, messes with his neighbors, and has a blatant disregard for direct requests." Darin argued constantly, even over the simplest issues. He always engaged in dialogue. His mother elaborated: "Yesterday he saw some cookies. I told him he needed to wait until lunch to eat them. He kept asking me about it for five minutes. Darin is quick to tell me when he perceives that something is unfair. If I say 'white,' he says 'black,' even when we discuss the littlest things. He'll be certain that he's right. It's very tiring for me. My child wants things his way and loses it if they're not. He breaks into tears at the drop of a hat."

Enthusiastic but impatient, Darin could not wait for things to happen. He demanded affection in an almost frantic, anxious way. His mother described it as a desperate feeling. He clung to her and did not want her to read or talk to anyone else. When he traveled, he fidgeted and pestered his brother. When he spent time with his dad, from whom his mother was divorced, he called his mother after only a few hours to complain that he missed her and wanted to go home.

Darin was anxious and insecure, fearful, but determined. He wanted to learn to ride his bicycle without training wheels from the very start. He was afraid of the dark and sleeping alone and had scary dreams.

When we asked Darin's mother about her pregnancy, she explained that she was very unhappy throughout the pregnancy. She felt frustrated and vulnerable about having to rely on Darin's father, who was irresponsible. She missed the security of having family around and kept fantasizing about moving to Hawaii to be with her parents.

We asked her whether Darin was more like her or his dad. Darin was very similar to his father, who didn't like to be by himself or to do things alone. Forever on the move, he was known for being a chronic procrastinator. Both father and son were reckless and accident-prone. Neither paid attention to where they were going.

Darin's only physical complaints were bumpy rashes on his hips and occasional headaches. His face was always pale, his ears red, and he had chronic puffiness under his eyes.

What was most unusual about Darin? His difficulty concentrating? His refusal to do what his mother asked? His unwillingness to settle down at night? Pestering his brother? All of these characteristics are very common in many children with ADHD. What really stood out in our eyes was Darin's oppositional nature, his strong response to being reprimanded or talked about, and the theme of homesickness in both Darin and in his mother. The medicine that best matches that combination of symptoms is *Capsicum* (red pepper). Again we gave Darin a single dose.

Darin's mother brought him back to see us two months later. "It was a gradual change. He's calmer. He's talking more and able to work things out better. My son's appetite is good and he's more willing to try new things. He's no longer asking if he's being good or quiet and there aren't as many arguments. He's more reasonable and rarely says the opposite. If I tell him he can't do something, he won't argue. He still pouts, but he gets over it easily. Maybe he's a little on the defiant side, but he becomes reasonable very quickly. There's been a gradual easing into being more agreeable. He's still impatient and sensitive to scolding and sad situations, but he's much more appropriate about demanding attention. Darin's also less clingy and possessive. He was unhappy for a few days about my starting to work, but now he's fine with it."

Darin had no more scary dreams. He had not talked about wanting to go home while visiting his father. His headaches were gone as well as the bumpy rashes on his hips. He continued to do quite well for over a year and did not need a repeat dose of the *Capsicum*. At that time the family moved to another state and continued home-opathic treatment locally.

"You're a Mean, Bad Mommy!"

Five-year-old Ben had sandy-brown hair, freckles, and a mischievous grin. His parents were at their wits' end when they brought him to us because of his extreme dis-obedience. Ben would not listen to his parents despite their efforts at numerous parenting techniques. When-ever his mother or father asked him to do something, he balked. There was absolutely no reasoning with him. If his parents warned, "You can't," he turned hysterical, screamed, cried, and threw whatever was in his vicinity. He engaged in slugging matches with his mother in pub-lic that embarrassed her terribly. He yelled, "I'm not afraid of you. It's not fair. You're a mean, bad mommy." Ben's defiance knew no limits.

Ben did not get along well with other children. He pushed and hit them, but when they did it back to him, he told them it was not fair. He liked to wrestle and play karate and insisted on taking charge whenever he played with other children. Ben was terrible with ani-mals. His parents had to tell him ten times a day to stop tormenting the cat and dog. It took Ben thirty to forty-five minutes to get dressed in the morning. He stopped and started over and over again and asked questions in-cessantly, driving his parents crazy.

Ben was a precocious child. He was bold and rel-ished climbing on high surfaces. He chattered for hours on end. Loud noises really bothered him. He was fixated on violence, weapons, and alien movies. Ben's moods could go from black to white in a matter of seconds, as if something snapped inside of him. When angry, he told his parents that he didn't want them to look at him or touch him. If others were injured, sometimes he was sympathetic and at other times he laughed. Ben talked very loudly and was extremely obstinate.

Ben complained of painful warts on his left foot and of growing pains. He was a restless sleeper and flailed his arms and legs in bed. He often woke upside down. He picked his nose and ground his teeth frequently. Ben loved noodles and sweets. He had an enormous appetite and often complained that he was "hungry to death."

We gave Ben a homeopathic medicine that is very useful for cross, irritable, contrary children who pick their noses and bottoms and grind their teeth. They are fussy, obstinate, throw tantrums, and do not want to be touched when mad. The medicine is derived from a plant named *Cina* (wormseed). These children sometimes have a history of pinworms or other parasites. Ben had a dramatic response to homeopathy. When his mother called six weeks after we gave him a dose of

Cina (wormseed)

Cross is the middle name of children needing *Cina*. They can be among the most irritable of children for no good reason. They do not seem to know what they want and reject what they are given. They want to be rocked but they do not like to be carried (except over the shoulder), touched, or looked at. They pinch, kick, and hit out of irritability and contradiction. Worms are a causative factor in some cases, especially pinworms. Children pick or bore into their nose or ears, scratch their bottoms, and grind their teeth at night. Serious cases may include convulsions.

Cina, she was delighted to report that the warts on the soles of his foot were completely gone. He had considerably decreased grinding his teeth. Most importantly, Ben's behavior was much better. "Now he's your normal, average kid." There had been no more slugging matches with his mom and no more temper tantrums. Ben was less defiant. To his mother's relief, he no longer told her that she was mean and bad. He also picked his nose much less. He was not as fixated on violence. His bones did not ache anymore. He did not complain about being touched. Ben needed one more dose of the *Cina* ten weeks later, then continued to do well. His noise sensitivity diminished considerably so that even a chain saw did not bother him.

Ben's mother gave birth to a second child five years later. She called us for help because of the baby's voracious appetite, shrieking, and fussiness. His little brother needed *Chamomilla,* a medicine quite similar to *Cina.*

Denise the Menace

Kaylie, a fourth-grader from New York, was a mischievous Denise the Menace-type little girl. She made it quite clear that she didn't like to clean her room and that she found her parents to be generally annoying. Especially when they started "talking, talking, talking" or they woke her up. Kaylie wore a sly grin on her face. This child had her moments. When asked to do something that wasn't on her preferred to-do list or when she perceived that her privacy had been invaded, Kaylie's modus operandi was to throw a tantrum. When out of sorts, she screamed and slammed her bedroom door and threw her stuffed animals across the room. Kaylie's father described her outbursts: "She blows up and becomes completely out of control. Kaylie shouts, 'I hate my life and everything in it!' She seems easily frustrated, even with the way her hair looks." This dramatic little girl had glaring, stomping, and rolling her eyes down to a fine art. Impatient and disgruntled, Kaylie was far too proud to admit her mistakes.

This young lady judged others harshly and was not one to cut them any slack. Her parents weren't the only ones who irritated her. Take her "former best friend," who had been mean to Kaylie. Or her teacher who, according to Kaylie, "gets mad at me and I get annoyed with her, too." An active, self-directed nine-year-old, Kaylie loved being in motion, particularly in the form of gymnastics, at which she excelled, although it took extra effort for her to build strength. A natural performer, she did her best while performing in front of others. "I'm the best at my gym!" she stated proudly. Kaylie could be a real tease and fooled people whenever she got a chance.

Kaylie was afraid of "big, fat, ferocious dogs," bees, being alone, falling asleep, and mountain roads. A night owl, she had a rough time going to bed at night and getting up in the morning. Her parents attributed this, in part, to her difficulty making transitions, which also included starting school after summer break.

Kaylie complained often of pain in her thighs, ankles, and knees, especially after a gymnastics workout. She also suffered periodic headaches and sore throats at bedtime. Kaylie's food favorites were pepperoni pizza, ice cream, candy, and fruit.

The medicine that Kaylie needed was quite clear from the start: *Calcarea phosphorica* (calcium phosphate). This medicine is a perfect fit for athletic, easily frustrated and annoyed, finicky kids who throw lots of temper tantrums. Kaylie's leg pain, fear of dogs and heights, and desire for smoked meat are also quite typical of children needing this medicine.

Five weeks after taking a dose of *Calcarea phosphorica*, Kaylie's parents informed us that she was having a better time at school and was less inclined towards anger and frustration. Her self-control was greater. At the four-month follow-up interview, Kaylie's mom was happy to say, "the amazing tantrums have not come back." Her knee and ankle pain was much improved, as was her overall strength.

Kaylie has received nine doses of the medicine over the past three and a half years. She has continued to progress quite nicely and has not needed any treatment for a little over a year.

A Button Pusher on Prozac

The earlier a child with ADHD begins homeopathy, the better. The right medicine can prevent years of social

Calcarea phosphorica (calcium phosphate)

Frustrated and dissatisfied are the two best words to describe many children needing *Calcarea phosphorica*. The grass is always greener for these kids, and they have that need to have or experience it. Cranky as toddlers, they can be hard to please. When they enter school, this is an excellent medicine for kids who become frustrated with their learning difficulties. School headaches and stomachaches as well as growing pains and fractures are common to children needing this medicine. They have a craving for sausage and smoked meat.

awkwardness, academic frustration, uncontrollable impulsivity, and damaged self-esteem. However, it is never too late to begin homeopathy. We first saw Dylan, a high-school student from eastern Oregon, when he was 16. "Dylan marches to his own beat," explained his mother. "His challenges with attention and obedience at school began when he was in the third grade. These problems led me to homeschool Dylan for the next three years. I tried him in a small, private school for a while in junior high school, but it didn't work out so I went back to homeschooling."

"We have a family history of depression and bipolar disorder. They've tried lots of different medications on Dylan, including lithium, but we only saw temporary improvements. Right now he's on Prozac. Dylan has a very sensitive, compassionate side. When he's good, he's really good. Then there's the other side of him—combative, aggressive, and outrageous. He loves to argue. Dylan has a genuine sense of justice and personal rights. Unfairness truly pushes his buttons."

Dylan had never been able to keep on track, make and follow through with plans, and organize his thoughts. He attributed it to his own laziness and lack of motivation and tells us that he just doesn't want to do things. Both Dylan and his dad were fascinated with ideas and loved to debate, especially about politics and Rush Limbaugh. Dylan didn't appreciate being hugged, touched, or mothered.

Although Dylan had his share of friends at school, he didn't get along with "the druggies and the goof-offs." They considered him a sitting duck and teased him whenever they found an opportunity. Although Dylan was not afraid to go against the crowd and prided himself on being different, he still didn't like being insulted. It made him extremely angry when other kids called him gay just to get him going. The more Dylan was criticized by the out crowd, the more he isolated himself.

Earlier in his life, Dylan had been hyperactive. He was much calmer now, though, by his own description, his favorite band was one that "made music for hyperactive kids." He still acted bizarrely from time to time to be funny, such as standing on the street carry signs with controversial or provocative slogans. Highly creative, he loved to build robots and compose songs. He had a dry, rather British, sense of humor.

Doing what he was told was not Dylan's strong suit. When asked to do anything, the most likely response was conflict, completing the task halfway, or not remembering to do it at all. Despite his own distaste for being teased, he heartily enjoyed provoking others to get a rise out of them. He could be downright disrespectful and confrontational with his siblings.

Dylan's parents had become so disgusted with him in recent months that they nearly asked him to move out. He refused to clean up after himself and was performing poorly in school. The recent return to homeschooling did bring up his grades from Ds to As and he was better able to track his assignments.

Hot-blooded, Dylan preferred to run around barefoot all year round. He didn't enjoy heat and preferred to sleep cool. He loved orange juice and olives.

The first and only medicine we have ever given Dylan is *Sulphur,* which matches his laziness, lack of motivation, desire to argue and debate, objection to injustice, difficulty concentrating, sloppiness, and his warm-blooded nature. Dylan slept more than usual over the first two to three weeks after taking the medicine, which can sometimes occur after taking a well-prescribed homeopathic medicine. Many positive changes ensued including considerably less combativeness and confrontation, greater amiability and cooperation, and a marked improvement in his grades. His level of anger had diminished, and he no longer admitted to any "sworn enemies." Dylan's symptoms returned to a lesser degree after he drank some coffee and the *Sulphur* was repeated. He was now taking the Prozac only at night. Impressed with Dylan's response to homeopathy, his parents chose to have him discontinue the Prozac at this point and he has never gone back to taking it.

Dylan has needed *Sulphur* six times over the past two and a half years, mainly due to his fondness for coffee. When he has needed a repetition, his attention span has shortened, and his impulsivity and disobedience have become more extreme, once to the point of his parents calling the sheriff because they couldn't get him to comply. With each dose of the *Sulphur,* his symptoms abated. Once his mom remarked on the tremendous change after the medicine, "from war to peace."

Now in his last year of high school, Dylan still needs a dose of *Sulphur* now and then. He knows he needs a dose when he feels less confident, uncomfortable socially, less witty, and prone to say "dumb things." Each time he takes the medicine, he responds very positively. Dylan is now thriving at school, holding two jobs at which he is excelling, and has no problems getting along with his family. He plans to attend community college next year. Dylan realizes how much better he feels when the *Sulphur* is acting and has chosen to avoid coffee so that each dose can last much longer.

16

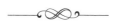

"I'm Gonna Chop Off His Head!"
ADHD with Violence and Rage

For four years, since *Ritalin-Free Kids* was first published, we have received calls almost daily from parents throughout the United States and overseas who have children with ADHD and other problems. A large number of the kids that we treated for ADHD, perhaps even half, also exhibit angry, aggressive, and violent behavior. Realizing what a significant difference homeopathic treatment could make in transforming rage into appropriate emotions and behavior, we wrote *Rage-Free Kids* to share the information more widely.[3] It was ironic and tragic that the 1999 Columbine massacre in Littleton, Colorado, occurred the day before we turned in our *Rage-Free Kids* manuscript.

More acts of violence have been perpetrated by and against children and adolescents than we could begin to mention in this book. We describe a few compelling cases to emphasize the importance of finding effective alternatives, such as homeopathy, to curb the epidemic

---

[3] Judyth Reichenberg-Ullman and Robert Ullman. *Rage-Free Kids.* Rocklin, CA: Prima, 1999.

of senseless violence in this country. First, from the foreword of *Rage-Free Kids:* "The threat of losing Nintendo apparently proved too much for a 12-year-old Edmonds [Washington] boy who was arrested Tuesday after he tried to choke his mother for taking away the controllers to his video game, police said. . . . She had gotten a report from his teacher that he'd failed to do his homework for several days and had been misbehaving in class. When she confronted him, he denied he had any homework, flew into a rage and attacked her, she reported. A similar incident occurred in Edmonds less than a year ago when a mother tried to take away her son's Sony PlayStation. The boy became angry and allegedly tried to strangle her."

A report documenting juvenile crime, "The Rise of the Young and the Ruthless," warned that America's children are turning to crime at such an alarming rate that juvenile arrests were likely to double by the year 2010. Juveniles were responsible for one out of every five violent crimes. Between 1983 and 1992, violations of juvenile weapons more than doubled for each racial group. From 1983 to 1992, the number of gun-related murders of juveniles increased fivefold. The authors found that one-quarter of juvenile victims were killed by other children. Finally, from 1980 to 1992, the number of children who were subjects of child abuse and neglect nearly tripled, from one million to almost three million children.[4]

Unfortunately, between the time of the first edition *Ritalin-Free Kids* in 1996 and of *Rage-Free Kids* three years later, violence still ran rampant. School violence, lockdowns, killings (both accidental and murders), and media violence in the form of television, movies, and video games continue to pervade our society. Guns

[4] *Seattle Times,* September 11, 1995, p. A5.

remain widely available. Clearly, this trend needs to be addressed at many different levels. For the individual aggressive child or adolescent, however, homeopathy can help, often dramatically, to turn around their minds and futures, and even, in some cases, to prevent future homicides or suicides.

These violent, even criminal, behaviors fall under the diagnostic category of Conduct Disorder, which is estimated to include 4–10 percent of children. The diagnosis is based on a violation of the basic rights of others and of age-appropriate societal norms.[5] "Conduct-disordered children exhibit a pattern of behavior that includes aggression, theft, vandalism, fire setting, opposition to authority, and other antisocial behaviors."[6] To be diagnosed with a conduct disorder, a child must have done at least three of the following for at least six months: stealing, running away, lying, arson, truancy, breaking and entering, destroying property, cruelty to animals or people, forced sexual activity, using a weapon in fights, and initiating fights. Teachers, counselors, and other parents often complain about these youngsters hurting others or behaving unacceptably, insolently, or even maliciously.

The good news is that homeopathic treatment *can* make a significant difference. We have found that in these children, anger masks or compensates for deeper feelings, most often fear, or even terror.

"I'm Gonna Kill You!"

Peter was a bubbly, blond seven-year-old boy. His Mariners sweatshirt and baseball cap fit the bill of a

[5] Schroeder and Gordon, op. cit., 280.
[6] Ibid., 280.

Little Leaguer. Peter's mom described him as "neurolog-
ically disorganized." "He didn't come out settled at
birth." Oversensitive to light and noise, Peter's system
just wasn't in synch. From birth, Peter cried constantly.
His only solace came from being rocked.

A loud talker, Peter's mood swings were severe,
like Jekyll and Hyde—sweet one minute, and threatening to kill the next. Frustrated in a flash of violent rage,
Peter kicked, hurled objects, bashed his toys, swore, and
talked repeatedly of murdering people. "I'm gonna get a
gun and shoot you. I'll hit you. I hate you," he menaced.
When younger, Peter bit other kids. When we first saw
him, his rages occurred at least twice a month; in earlier
years, they happened several times a week.

This was only one side of Peter. The other side was
sweet, intelligent, and wouldn't want to hurt a fly. Peter
lamented to his mother, "I'm really stupid, dumb. Help
me stop doing this!" But he lacked the self-restraint to
stop himself. The child was also an incredible actor and
singer and created a rich fantasy world.

Peter's concentration was "all over the map." He
was up and down in his chair. At school Peter engaged
in frequent skirmishes with other children. Terrified of
the dark and of dogs, he was also afraid to put his head
under water. Peter had recurrent nightmares about monsters trying to get him, leading him to scream out in the
middle of the night.

What struck us the most about Peter was the violence of his responses. Whether fear or rage, Peter responded to the world as if he were in immediate danger
and must respond accordingly to defend himself. This
violence and the numerous fears, especially of dogs,
monsters, and the water, are classic for the medicine
Stramonium. The eruption of anger in people needing

this medicine seems to reflect unconscious, raw, animal instincts. These people tend to feel as if they are alone in the forest surrounded by dangerous wild animals and must be on guard at every moment, particularly in the dark.

Peter's mother noticed the difference in him within three days after he took *Stramonium*. He was much sweeter. There were no more rages. He was very co-operative and helpful and seemed happier overall. Peter was more tenacious with his reading and more willing to push himself. He no longer talked about killing any-one. His anger was one-tenth of what it was before the homeopathy.

Peter was overall much improved from the *Stramonium*. He did not mention anything at all about killing

Stramonium
(*Datura stramonium* or thorn apple)

Children matching the picture of *Stramonium* ex-hibit a mixture of extreme fear and violence. The feeling is like the terror of being in a dark jungle surrounded by wild animals that may attack them at any moment, and the response is violence and rage. These children are very afraid of the dark, es-pecially when alone, and can become extremely clingy. They may become violent if provoked. They fear animals, water, and violent death. They often have nightmares or terrors with shrieking. Stammering, cursing, jealousy, and rage are com-mon behaviors. These are very intense children. A very frightening or traumatic event such as violent abuse or birth trauma may catapult a child into a *Stramonium* state.

anyone until one year later, at which time we increased the strength of the medicine. He has needed a total of five doses of the medicine over two-and-a-half years.

Suspended from Kindergarten!

Antonio's mom first called us from Idaho when he was eight. The family was disturbed by his inconsolable tantrums over the least little thing like having his sandwich sliced in the wrong direction or pulling the plug on the bathtub at the wrong time. Antonio's aggressive behavior first surfaced in kindergarten, when he began to hit, bite, and cream other kids in the head with whatever ball was at hand. In fact Antonio was actually suspended from kindergarten for attempting to strangle a classmate.

Diagnosed with ADHD in the first grade, Antonio was given Ritalin. The medication gave a boost to his focus, but did nothing for his aggression and tendency to burst into tears at the least provocation. He was again suspended from school for fighting on the playground. Antonio's mom mentioned at this point that his father had likewise not been a person who avoided challenges. A rock climber and skydiver, his father had been killed in a motorcycle accident while Antonio was in his mother's womb. He, too, was one bright, tough cookie and was kicked out of school for fighting. His father's death was a tremendous shock to his mom, and she had second thoughts about whether she could handle a child on her own.

Second grade, his mother continued, brought yet another suspension for—again—combative behavior toward a peer. Antonio was not intimidated by age or authority. Disrespectful to adults and children alike, he was well known for his smart mouth and considered himself as the equal of everyone. This kid would argue with anybody over anything. At times his outbursts were triggered by someone hurting his feelings or antagonizing him, but he didn't really need anyone else to get the action going. Now, in third grade, he was as feisty as ever.

Eccentric, highly gifted, and brilliant, Antonio loved using big words and was extremely articulate. "I'm spoiled," Antonio said. "I want my own way all the time. My grandparents fuss over me because I'm adorable. You know what's on my bulletin board? Bill Clinton, a sawtooth shark trying to devour a goldfish, and a photo of me that says 'Am I cute or what?' " Antonio was not particularly athletic nor did he thrive in groups. He lost it at family reunions. Antonio and his stepdad got along very well together, although, when disciplined, he would inevitably shout, "You're not my real father."

His precocious and articulate nature made Antonio a wonderful child to interview. "I wasn't very friendly last year," he confided, "because I had to get up way too early. That made me grumpy. If someone even bumped into me without apologizing, it would make me want to fight. I'm really sensitive feeling-wise. Especially when kids tease me about my glasses. Or if they call me a name or play a nasty joke on me. I just think we're all equal."

"I get good grades. Reading is my best subject. Art is next. I read plays, stories, fairy tales, and folk tales. And I love science. And insects! My teacher tells us all about red and black ants. I like every subject but math. I just don't get addition and subtraction. I'm not going to college. I plan to start my career early. As an architect. You know, I design things right in my very own house. Like a future railroad on a cylindrical track with a hole cut through it connected with invincible chains and poles. I even built a restaurant with my Lego's."

Hershey's chocolate and coffee-flavored shakes were Antonio's favorites, with pizza and Rice Dream close behind. He was also a fan of Italian and Chinese food, particularly hot-and-sour soup.

Homeopathic *Tungsten* and *Angustura* produced no change in Antonio. *Veratrum album,* prescribed several months later when Antonio began to kiss and hug other kids inappropriately, resulted in a partial improvement. After seven months of treatment, we gave Antonio *Sulphur,* the most commonly prescribed of all homeopathic medicines, but not one we have prescribed much for aggressive children. The prescription finally became clear when Antonio emphasized his defensiveness and overreaction to being teased or criticized. At this point, Antonio's mom commented that she, too, felt terribly teased as a child, although never aggressive. His mother went on to share that she, too, was precocious and had to have the last word. *Sulphur* fit the precocity, eccentricity, defiance, quarrelsomeness, and Antonio's way with words. Antonio's sloppiness, inventive mind, and sensitivity to the odors of others, combined with his obliviousness to how *he* smelled, confirmed the prescription of *Sulphur.*

At his six-week follow-up visit, we could see some change. More willing to cooperate, Antonio was much less prone to fly off the handle. The incidence of arguing at home diminished, and he now apologized after behaving unacceptably. He still had gotten in trouble twice—once for spitting on other children and another time for hitting them.

At his next appointment, his mother reported that the daily behavior evaluations from school had been consistently positive. For the most part, he was more compliant. Antonio assured us, "My days of hitting are past. I throw words around now instead of punches."

School continued to go well with no further reports of problematic behavior, despite the death of his stepfather. Antonio's grades were fine and he no longer fought with his peers. "I've had a pretty neutral life," he confided, "pretty routine and boring." When doing something that held no interest for him, Antonio found his mind to be "like a cloud driven by the wind." He continues to do much better despite throwing an occasional sand bomb or eraser at someone he doesn't like.

During our last visit, Antonio told us all about parabolic dish radiation reflectors that emitted curved light, melted the desired target, and were able to produce more energy. He also shared with us how he was in the process of designing a huge spaceship that could travel to all corners of the galaxy, wherever it happened to be needed. His ship had a crew of nine, a special generator, and was surrounded by a force-field warp bubble "that makes you smaller than half the size of a light particle."

Homeopathy has helped Antonio harness his energy and kept his argumentativeness in check. One of the complaints we hear from parents about Ritalin and other stimulant medications is that they dampen children's innate creativity. Clearly, Antonio continues to be a highly spirited, advanced thinking, mischievous child, yet his behavior is now socially acceptable.

"Everything He Does Is Too Intense"

Kirk's mother knew nothing about homeopathy, but she had read one of our articles about homeopathic treatment of ADHD and was willing to try almost anything to civilize her son. Kirk, age seven, had tried all of the ADHD medications, each of which caused side effects. The most recent one, an antidepressant, had resulted in blinking eyes, shoulder shrugs, and tics. Kirk's mother described him wearily: "He bugs people; he's in their face. He just can't settle down or concentrate. He moves at such a fast pace. It's irritating. In groups, he's always the bad guy. He can't wait for his turn. When he gets mad, he slugs and kicks. He's all-around obnoxious. Kirk's impulsive. He has to have everything right now. He even pulls out his loose teeth before they fall out. He never thinks about the consequences."

Kirk's mom homeschooled him, as is typical with many of the children in our practice. He found math easy, but he still could not read. He had a hard time remembering what he learned.

Power and control were vital to Kirk. His family lived on a farm, and he loved to chase the chickens and ride the calf. When he got mad, Kirk became very destructive. He hurled his toys and stomped on them. Kirk held grudges and was unforgiving of anyone who wronged him. He had absolutely no remorse when he hurt others. Tripping others was good sport.

Kirk's mother continued, "Everything he does is too intense. He runs over his baby sister without thinking. He hits his siblings then smirks and says they deserved it. Seeing others get into trouble is exciting to him. He pesters his brother and sisters and just won't quit." Kirk was "tender with a hard shell." His self-esteem was low. He felt that nobody loved him.

Kirk had been a perfect angel until he was three, when his sister was born. He would hold the baby by the neck. His mother feared that he would strangle his sister and would not let him carry her. Once he struck her. Another time he stuck his finger down her throat.

Terrified of the dark, Kirk needed to have his mother by his side at night. He hated loud noises and used to cry when he heard fireworks or the lawn mower. He had night terrors when he was younger.

Kirk still was not potty trained; he had never been dry at night and had some wet spots during the day. He also complained of headaches "like someone is really pounding my head."

We prescribed *Stramonium* for Kirk because of his violent tendencies. At his four-month follow-up, Kirk's mother described how he had improved in every area and that the tics, which remained from the antidepressant, were gone. "Now he's sensitive. He even picked a flower for me yesterday. Before he didn't even have a conscience. He trips other kids now only if they provoke him."

Kirk's behavior continued to improve on the *Stramonium*. He needed a dose of the medicine on an average of once every three months. Generally one dose of a homeopathic medicine lasts four to six months or longer.

Two and a half years after beginning treatment, Kirk's mother felt that the *Stramonium* was no longer working well. At this time she provided more details about her son's behavior. His arguments with his sister began with verbal battering and lack of cooperation, then escalated into kicking, punching, and hair pulling. It was a matter of power and control.

What disturbed his mother the most about Kirk was his complete lack of compassion and remorse. When his baby sister got her finger slammed in the car door, he did not offer to help. Kirk and some other boys got into a rock-throwing fight at the church barbecue. When his rock hit another child in the eye, he seemed pleased and told his mom it was the other boy's fault.

Kirk's mom recounted to us for the first time his experience with BBs the year before. He shot a bird in the air, a goat in the udder, and the family's pet cat. He lied and told his parents their pet dog attacked the cat. When his father threatened to shoot the dog, Kirk still did not admit to what he had done. When they took the cat to the vet, they found the BBs. Kirk acted as if he had done nothing wrong.

Kirk's total lack of conscience was very striking. He was intentionally malicious toward others, and when they were hurt he showed absolutely no remorse. We could only imagine where this would lead Kirk as an adult if his behavior remained unchecked. This type of meanness with a lack of any conscience led us to give Kirk a medicine for people who care little about others, isolate themselves, build up a store of tremendous anger, then strike out in a cruel, even inhuman, way. They may even become so savagely enraged that they kill someone without regret. They lack the moral conscience that is the guiding principle for most members of society. This substance is *Scorpion.*

Three months after we prescribed *Scorpion* for Kirk, his mother reported a distinct improvement. Instead of hurting his siblings when he became angry, he would now walk away. He was helping them more and being more protective. He was no longer physically aggressive. Time-outs, which were previously futile, now worked well with Kirk. His attention and attitude had

Scorpion (androctonos)

The scorpion lives under rocks in the desert and
stings its prey to death by sudden attacks. Children
who need *Scorpion* lack a conscience and compassion for the suffering of others. They can be extremely violent, hurting or even murdering others
if provoked or just for the fun of it. Parents of these
children often fear bodily harm or that their children are headed for a life of criminal violence.
These children are detached from other people
and like to be alone, removed from the demands
of society, as though they are viewing the world
distantly through a small hole in the rocks. They
are absolutely self-centered. Indifferent to pleasure
or pain, to others' opinion of them, and to any du-
ties or responsibilities, they live in self-imposed
isolation.

also improved. Kirk's mother concluded, "He's nicer.
We can live with him." He has needed intermittent repetitions of the *Scorpion*. When he relapses, he turns into
a different person, one whom his mother despises, and
she calls us immediately for help. Fortunately we treat
Kirk's mother and siblings, which has made it somewhat easier for the whole family to cope with Kirk.

We Call Him "Mad Brandon"

Brandon's mother called us from Oklahoma with great
hope that we could help her family. "I saw your book at
the health food store, and homeopathy sounded like just
what we were looking for. You're treating my son today,

me later this week, and, if all goes well, my husband in a couple of months. We're committed!"

"Brandon was a handful from the start—fussy, hard to please, hungry all the time. At three months, he was hospitalized for a febrile illness, which tested negative for meningitis, and given intravenous antibiotics. A colicky infant, Brandon was not one for cuddling and never seemed satisfied. By the time he was two, we could tell that he was overactive and avoided eye contact and group play with other children." Highly sensitive, Brandon would throw a fit whenever his parents took him to the barbershop for a haircut. His father had to hold him down the entire time. Because the parents were concerned that Brandon wasn't talking even after he turned two, their family doctor recommend that he have his hearing evaluated. This was impossible without sedation because of Brandon's refusal to have his head touched.

High fevers of 102 to 103 Fahrenheit were frequent for Brandon. As a baby, he would tense up, as if he experienced pain in the back of his neck and spine, whenever his mom tried to burp him. He cried constantly all day, his face turned red and his eyes glassy, and he was easily disturbed by any abrupt movement around his body. Brandon's grandfather was much the same. Nicknamed "Mad Sam," no one could ever get close to him. Like Brandon, he hated loud noises, having his head or face touched, and everyone had to walk on eggshells around him. Needless to say, nobody liked Sam. And he was bitter until the day he died at eighty-eight.

Brandon was now four, and although he and his parents had survived toddlerhood, he was still a ball of fire. Going to bed was a battle—Brandon shrieked, flew into a rage, pulled at his clothes, and "flashed his eyes like a caged animal." He detested being confined. Mad Brandon crossed his arms, locked his feet together, lowered his head, slumped his head, turned his back, and growled. If the family dogs barked, so did Brandon. He crawled on the ground, drank out of their water bowls, savored dog and cat food, and joined the dogs when they chased the chickens. The minute he got home, Brandon ripped off his clothes and ran around the house "buck-naked."

"Brandon's a guy on the go. Strong willed, a skilled manipulator, and really good-looking. He knows it, too. Quite the charmer. He's drawn to rough play and thrill rides. Once he gets his mind set on something, he just won't let go. Brandon will eat just one thing for weeks and watch the same video, like *Thomas the Tank Engine* or *Star Wars,* over and over again for weeks. "

"Our son has a hard time separating from us and lately, he's fought going to school. He got down from the school bus when he wasn't supposed to, then took off running after it when he realized what he'd done. He loves to control at home or at school. A born leader, he demands that the rest of the class does as he instructs. Brandon is in a federally funded school for kids with behavioral or leaning problems or handicaps."

"Being at home with Brandon is no piece of cake. He won't tolerate a babysitter, so we've been prisoners of our own home. It's impossible to take him out in public because of his meltdowns. He screams bloody murder, stands in place and kicks, kicks doors if we start to walk out without him, and, recently, he's taken to hitting us."

"The odd thing is that he seems to be aware of what he's going through, but is powerless to stop himself. When he's sweet and everything is going well, Brandon is a model child. He laughs in his sleep and, when we try to wake him, his tongue gets stuck on the roof of his mouth. When Brandon hears organ music, he melts into a puddle of tears. There's no telling what he's going to do next!"

Full of fears, Brandon was terrified of the dark and thunderstorms, and came unglued if even a drop of water touched him, in which case every piece of clothing had to be removed. He wouldn't even get his feet wet. This little fellow insisted on lukewarm or cold food or drinks, except when he became overheated in the summer and went for ice cream. Brandon wouldn't get anywhere near a hot bath.

Brandon fit the picture of *Belladonna:* high fevers, hypersensitivity to noise, touch, and heat, desire to escape, shrieking, tantrums, and a fear of water, the dark, and storms. Two months later, his mother happily reported that Brandon was much easier to work with, his outbursts were no longer traumatic, he was now reachable, and, to her relief, he finally seemed to have a conscience. Typical of children who receive the correct homeopathic medicine, he experienced an immediate growth spurt. Brandon had moved up to the top class in his community school, and his speech had improved dramatically. It was a if "a light bulb went on." Before homeopathic treatment, he had resisted doing his ABCs and counting. Not anymore. The director of school is seeing no evidence of ADHD and plans to transition him to regular school next fall. They tell us now that his learning is excellent."

"Our extended family noticed the difference in Brandon immediately—that he was much more directed. When they told him it was time for him to go home, there wasn't his usual meltdown. Now Brandon is much more affectionate, tells us how much he loves us, and apologizes appropriately. We no longer need to cut all the tags off of his clothes, and he doesn't bark like a dog. Nor was he growling or sharing food and water with the dogs or chasing the chickens. His bedwetting has improved greatly. Brandon's cheeks aren't red like they used to be, and his sleep is somewhat better."

Brandon was still quick to correct and debate his parents and continued to "argue with the fence post." His previously low pain threshold was now normal; he no longer fought over going to bed, no longer had the flashing eyes of a caged animal, and was not as strongly affected by loud noises. Getting his feet wet didn't bother him anymore, he was much happier about going to school, and he had stopped kicking doors and screaming.

Three months after taking the first dose of *Belladonna,* the bedwetting had stopped entirely, and the overall improvement persisted. Six months later, Brandon was calmer, had a longer fuse, and his attitude at home and at school was significantly better. His parents report that he is now much happier, sleeps well, no longer barks or fights about every little thing, and has become much more creative. "We're able to be so much more patient with Brandon. It's a miracle." It helped considerably that both of his parents have also experienced a dramatic improvement in their own health with homeopathic treatment. The new and improved Brandon recently graduated from preschool, complete with cap and gown!

"Girls Can Be Violent, Too"

Rachel struck us as intense from the moment she walked into our office. She had bright red (dyed) hair, a look-you-right-in-the-eyes gaze, and a certain determination about her. She had recently been caught shoplifting. She habitually lied. Her behavior had been violent since she was very small. She became so self-destructive that she mutilated herself, scratched her face deeply, hit her head, and pulled out her hair "in gobs."

Rachel told us, "There are a lot of people who hate me. They're always calling me bad names, making fun of me, and saying that they hate me. I just hate it. Ever since I started going to school it's been like that. Everywhere I go there are people who hate me. They just say bad stuff. They call me a robber. They called me that the whole time on the bus. I try to ignore them."

Her mother elaborated. Rachel used to lash out at people verbally and create a major crisis. She screamed repeatedly in elementary school and would not calm down. She hit her mother when she felt her mother was reprimanding her. Kicking and punching were everyday responses for her. Sometimes Rachel pushed her mother just for talking too loudly. Rachel generally felt bad after her rages and apologized.

Rachel threatened to hurt herself with a knife a couple of months before we first saw her. When she felt very angry toward her mother, the more her mother talked to her, the more deeply she would scratch her own face. When Rachel hit hard, she often said, "I'm bad. I'm stupid. I shouldn't be alive." She picked up cats when they tried to run away. She bugged her little kitten to get a rise out of her. Rachel had a hard time concentrating. She became easily overwhelmed but could "go into another land where she didn't hear things."

We asked Rachel's mother about her pregnancy, since the state of the mother during pregnancy often provides valuable clues to the homeopath about the state of the child and about which medicine is needed.

Rachel's parents argued continually during the pregnancy. Her father was emotionally violent and controlling. He frequently yelled and swore and would occasionally break and throw things. Long contractions during the pregnancy frightened Rachel's mother. She was given Demerol for the pain, and Rachel was delivered by suction extraction.

Rachel's mother described her as a "Buddha baby": bald, happy, and interested in life. Her behavior changed when she was four years old and was molested by a five-year-old girl at her preschool. She would never say much about that experience to her mother except to say that the other little girl made her do things she did not want to do.

She was afraid of the dark when she was younger and still kept the night-light on in case she woke up disoriented in the middle of the night. She also feared big, vicious dogs and was afraid they would "jump out and bite" her head off. Her fear of dogs was exacerbated by the "cat-killing dogs" that would bark at her when she got off the school bus. When she was three, Rachel was bitten on the face by a dog after she teased him. When her mother thought more about when Rachel's behavior became violent, and she realized that the change coincided with the dog bite.

Accident-prone, Rachel tripped on a regular basis, suffered "a bazillion" contusions and abrasions, broke her wrist in a bicycle accident, and broke her knuckle twice, once punching a wall and another time hitting another child. She pulled a tendon in her thumb a different time, twice experienced eraser burns, and had casts four or five times for various injuries.

She used to be terrified of vampires under her bed. She dreamed that vampires came in and bit everyone in her family. Then the vampires ran away and hid under her bed. She ultimately lost her fear after dreaming about little vampire bugs on skateboards. The dream made her laugh, and the fear dissipated.

We prescribed *Lyssin,* a medicine made from the saliva of a rabid dog, that matched Rachel's fits of animal-like rage, complete with scratching, screaming, cutting, and kicking. Her history of abuse and her feeling of being teased to the point of torment fit the picture of the medicine very well, as did her rage with quick repentance, her fear of dogs and vampires, and, last but not least, her violent behavior began soon after she was bitten in the face by a dog. Another contributing factor was the violent anger of her father and the arguments between her parents while she was in utero.

Five days after Rachel took the *Lyssin,* her mother wrote us a letter reporting quite a dramatic change in

Lyssin (rabies nosode)

The main feeling in those fitting the *Lyssin* state is torment followed by rage, like a dog who has been kicked and abused over and over and finally bites its master. This medicine may be useful in cases of child abuse, particularly sexual abuse. The *Lyssin* rage is followed rapidly by apologies. These children are among the most violent and difficult to handle. Sometimes there is a history of a dog bite or being scared by a dog. Fears of water and dogs are prominent, as is claustrophobia. There is often an impulse to cut oneself or others. These children may be aggravated by the sound or sight of running water. Bedwetting may be a problem.

her daughter. She told us, "It's sort of like the Buddha infant delight in the world is returning along with a heightened ability to incorporate the rigors of the world as 'normal' experiences."

Rachel has continued to do remarkably well since we began treating her. Initially she had better conscious control over her outbursts, and her violent episodes became infrequent. She became less accident-prone almost immediately. Within three months, Rachel was having only little tantrums. Throwing and kicking things were as bad as her violent behavior became. She now had friends, for whom she bought Christmas presents. She was having "a whole bunch of good, strange dreams" rather than her nightmares of the past, and her sleep was much improved. She was doing much better in school, getting all A's and B's except for a C+ in math. Her grades just preceding homeopathic treatment included an F in physical education and a D in math. She stopped the shoplifting and face scratching. She still occasionally felt the urge to hurt herself, but now she hit herself with something soft instead of cutting herself.

Nine months after starting homeopathy, Rachel was doing wonderfully. She had experienced no angry outbursts. She had not broken anything in a long time, or even thrown or kicked anything and no longer hit herself. Her grades continued to be very good. Rachel had just learned that she would be transferred out of a special-needs classroom into a regular classroom in the fall. She felt much better about herself, had no significant violent outbursts, and was no longer accident-prone. Rachel's mom has also done extremely well with homeopathic treatment. Their relationship is much better than it was prior to homeopathy.

As we wrote up Rachel's case for our book, we were struck by her mother's description of the change in her daughter after being on the medicine for one week. She used the word "delightful." That is the same word that had come into our minds in describing our interactions with Rachel now. She really is a delight.

17

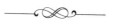

"Won't I Ever Outgrow This?"
Adults with ADHD

The prevalence of ADHD among adults is estimated at 2 to 7 percent of the adult population.[3] We have noticed that some of the children brought to us for ADHD are carbon copies of one or both of their parents. The mother often reports, "Billy's just like his dad. He can't pay attention to save his life. I have to ask him questions six times, just like Billy." Or she might report that, although his dad has grown out of his ADHD traits, as a child, he got into trouble for the exact same things Billy is doing now.

You may have concluded that you have ADHD after one or more of your children has received the diagnosis or after reading a piece about the disorder in the popular media about someone who sounds just like you. You may have experienced a revelation as you finally found a label to explain why you had such a hard time as a child and adult following the program and fitting into the mold of "normality." *Driven to Distraction*, written by two candid and knowledgeable psychiatrists who personally admit to having ADHD, has turned many an

---

[3] Paul H. Wender, *Attention Deficit Hyperactivity Disorder in Adults* (New York/Oxford: Oxford University Press, 1995).

adult on to the idea that they or their partner may have ADHD.[4]

Exactly how many kids with ADHD grow up to be adults with ADHD is debatable. Some researchers have concluded that the prevalence of ADHD declines exponentially with age and that the rate of ADHD in a given age group seems to decline by 50 percent every five years.[5] As few as 4 percent of adults who had been diagnosed with ADHD were found to still have the disorder at the age of twenty-four;[6] however, two-thirds of twenty-five year-old patients who had been hyperactive as children still complained of at least one symptom of ADHD (and that symptom could affect their lives significantly).[7] Usually adults suffer less from the climbing-the-walls restlessness and ignore-the-consequences impulsivity of kids with ADHD, although even these unnerving traits may persist into adulthood in some cases. A number of the parents of children whom we treat for ADHD do in fact complain that some of the traits have lingered into adulthood. Fortunately, it is never too late to begin homeopathic treatment for ADHD. Adults with ADHD experience can suffer such severe inattention and lack of focus that routine desk jobs may

---

[4] Edward Hallowell and John Ratey, *Driven to Distraction: Recognizing and Coping with Attention Deficit Disorder from Childhood Through Adulthood* (New York: Pantheon Books, 1994).

[5] J.D. Hill, and E.P. Schoener, "Age-dependent Decline of Attention-deficit Hyperactivity Disorder." *American Journal of Psychiatry* 153: 1143–1146 (1996).

[6] S. Mannuaaz, R.G. Klein, A. Bessler, P. Malloy, and M. La Padula, "Adult Psychiatric Status of Hyperactive Boys Grown Up." *American Journal of Psychiatry* 155: 493–498 (1998).

[7] G. Weiss and L.T. Hechtman, *Hyperactive Children Grown Up: ADHD in Children, Adolescents, and Adults* (New York: Guildford Press, 1993).

seem impossible and, despite a high level of intelligence, they may be perceived as chronic underachievers. Highly distractible, they often need frequent reminders to complete tasks, and still may never get around to doing so. Off in another world, these individuals may or may not hear what is said to them, and family, friends, and coworkers may feel as if they are not fully present and accounted for. Forgetting where they put their keys, purse, airline ticket, or will; confusing or entirely missing appointments; or misplacing or forgetting to pay bills lead these people to appear irresponsible, even though they might actually be overly conscientious in an attempt to compensate. Disorganization, absentmindedness, procrastination, and wishful thinking are typical. ADHD is not synonymous with decreased intelligence or mental capacity. In fact, people with ADHD can be geniuses and excel in their field, as was the case with Winston Churchill, who was told he would never succeed. Individuals with ADHD can become inventors, scientists, philosophers, artists, or neurosurgeons—their minds soar while others pick up the pieces of their everyday lives so they can function in the real world.

Adults with ADHD, like children, may be clumsy and awkward with social skills that do not match their intellects. The impulsivity and compromised judgment of childhood ADHD that leads one to jump off a roof or climb a high beam may turn into reckless driving, playing the futures market, risky sexual practices, or any other form of dangerous behavior. These grownups may exhibit tremendous restlessness, just as they did as kids, flitting from one job, task, or idea to the next. They may either thrive on or crumble under the pressure of stress or overstimulation.

Who Has Time to Sleep?

Carl came to see us at age thirty-seven. Frightened by a strong family history of cancer, he hoped we could strengthen his immune system and increase his chances of avoiding cancer. Carl suffered from congenital hearing loss, also a family trait.

"I tend to work on a crisis basis. I procrastinate and do everything inefficiently. My family is riddled with cancer: my father, mother, and lots of other relatives have had cancer. Preventive medicine doesn't always fit into my lifestyle. I've always had convenient excuses. I like to think of myself as quite easygoing, but I must admit that stress affects me. I rebel against others' expectations by procrastinating. Then I feel ashamed when I fall short of their expectations. I berate myself because I'm lazy."

Carl had a history of compulsive drinking and recreational drugs use. A man of excess, once Carl started anything, he just could not quit. He enjoyed engaging in sex as often as possible and masturbated frequently. He had a history of venereal warts as well as herpes on the mouth and canker sores. We noticed that Carl fidgeted incessantly during the interview.

A software programmer, Carl described his concentration as "almost hypnotic in focus" and his memory as extremely good, yet his follow-through was sporadic. It was all or nothing with Carl. He had no clue how to pace himself. When he listened to a song, he felt compelled to play it over and over again. A heavy-duty partier in college, he got into the habit of working all night. He worked regularly up to forty-eight hours straight without sleeping, then napped for six hours to catch up before beginning the cycle again. Carl's perfect schedule was to stay up until 2 or 3 A.M. and sleep until 10 or 11 A.M. the next day. "I've never been a morning person. Only under duress will I get up."

He was also excessive in his eating habits. Sour foods and key lime pie were his favorites. The more sour the taste, the better he liked it. As a child, Carl loved taking a jar of lemon juice out of the refrigerator and mixing it with sugar to make a sour paste. He also had a strong desire for Granny Smith apples, really tart and crisp, as well as salty foods and buttermilk. Carbonated soft drinks were Carl's beverage of choice.

Recurrent sinus problems and hay fever bugged Carl. A serious teeth grinder, he wondered if this habit might be a reflection of anger that he held within instead of expressing it to those who expected things of him. Carl was fearless. He enjoyed taking chances and doing things other people might perceive as risky.

We gave Carl a homeopathic nosode called *Medorrhinum*. What stood out most the intensity with which he did everything. Driven to do everything to excess, there was no middle of the road for Carl. He was either in high gear or at a standstill. We also prescribed this medicine for him because of his restless, erratic temperament. Carl had an intensity that was striking, even after we talked with him for just a few minutes. Life was a series of one intense experience after another. People needing this medicine often have very poor follow-through, as Carl described. They may have severe memory problems, though Carl did not, as well as a compulsive bent, history of warts, and a strong desire for sour foods and salt.

At his first return visit six weeks later, Carl reported that he had felt moodier and more short-tempered for the first two days following the homeopathic treatment, then noticed an increase in his dandruff and teeth clenching for two weeks. He then found himself waking at six in the morning regardless of when he went to sleep. He experienced a burst of productivity and had accomplished a great deal.

Two months later, Carl reported that his mind was clear and fast. He was not procrastinating as much. He no longer waited until the last minute to write papers. He was engaged in more long-range planning. He was no longer staying up as late. He was in bed now by 1 A.M. instead of 2 or 3. His warts disappeared completely. He had a new girlfriend with whom he had a very active sexual relationship and he no longer felt the urge to masturbate.

Homeopathic treatment continued to help Carl, except when he resorted to recreational drugs, which interfered with the treatment. Over the two-and-one-half years of treatment, homeopathy helped him to channel his energy in more positive directions. Carl became more able to deal with others' expectations openly and honestly. He stopped pretending he had done something

Medorrhinum (nosode)

The minds of these folks race a mile a minute, their minds crowded with a thousand thoughts at once. Night owls, these kids can stay up till all hours then want to sleep in the following morning. Passionate children and adults, they crave extremes of experience anywhere and anytime they can get it. Memory can be a real problem. They may bite their fingernails, or even toenails, to the quick. Diaper rash, sinusitis, warts, asthma, and arthritis are typical physical problems. Those needing *Medorrhinum* often love oranges, unripe fruit, ice, sweets, salt, and fat.

that he had not, which had gotten him into lots of trouble before. His excessive approach to life diminished, and he finally established a moderate pace for himself.

"I Feel Like I'm Jumping Out of My Skin"

At age 25, superachiever Jill sought out homeopathic care due to "nervous symptoms." She had always felt nervous and hurried. It was an internal feeling that others often did not notice. "There's an awful lot that I can't get done. I become tense and feel like I'm gonna jump right out of my skin. I get hot. It feels like a hot flash, an adrenaline rush. When I feel nervous, I get weak in the knees and experience sloshy, gurgling sensation in my abdomen accompanied by diarrhea. I was diagnosed with colitis three years ago, but I had the beginnings of an ulcer at nineteen."

Jill felt jumpy about her family and about keeping up with life. She had raised her young son as a single mom while taking a full-credit load at the university and graduated Phi Beta Kappa cum laude with a degree in physical therapy. A highly responsible person, she worried obsessively about what she needed to do. Jill often became nervous to the point of hyperventilating and her fingers turned blue. It was hard for her to relax unless she was exhausted or sick. She remembered enjoying having the flu as a child so she could relax. Jill's worry-wart nature came early. At her third birthday party, she remembered that her birthday wish was that the stock market would go up because she was worried about the family finances. Jill's nickname as a child was "Chatterbox." Her mother trained her not to bother people. It was hard for Jill to keep her hands off of the other girls' curly hair and to avoid touching things in stores.

She complained of a heightened sensitivity to her environment. Jill felt oversensitive to music, weather, and to feelings inside a room. Not much escaped her. She had an exaggerated startle response and reflexes. It was as if she were always ready to explode. She became so angry at times that it scared her. She used to be a heavier drinker. Once when drunk, she tried to choke her ex-husband.

Jill was constantly "fighting against a busy depression." "I have to stay busy. I'm not good at home unbusy. I'd like to feel more comfortable with myself doing nothing. I have the urge to touch people, arm wrestle, put my hands on their heads, but I hold myself back because of social rules. I think about it all the time. I have impulses to kiss people I don't know, but I don't allow myself to act on them. I rarely meet a couple that I don't imagine in bed together. My mind is full of socially unacceptable thoughts."

Her mother told Jill that people wouldn't like her if she were fat; she developed a history of anorexia and bulimia. She became very involved in athletics in junior high school. Already a mere size four or five dress size, Jill began to binge and starve. Laxative binges were routine from age nineteen to twenty-two. She suffered from painful menstrual cramps. She had nightmares about being responsible for too much and disappointing others. Jill craved bread. During her pregnancy, she often peeled lemons and ate them whole. She still loved sour lemonade, grapefruit, and pickles. She got diarrhea from whole milk or ice cream.

What made Jill most memorable was her perpetual need to keep busy, busy, busy, quite a bit different from the all-or-nothing approach of Carl. The two share the characteristic of restlessness and high sexual energy, but their life experience is very different. Jill had to be touching, kissing, talking. She was compelled to be doing something every minute of her life.

We chose *Veratrum album* (white hellebore) for Jill because of her internal restlessness, impulse to touch and kiss others, hurriedness, tendency to menstrual cramps, diarrhea from dairy products, and her strong craving for sour foods. We saw her again three months later. She reported feeling much better beginning one week after she took the medicine. She told us, "My stomach hasn't felt this good since I was twenty years old. I didn't even remember how good it could feel. I am so much more relaxed. The restlessness and hurriedness are much better and so is my hypersensitivity to the environment." Since receiving the two doses of *Veratrum,* Jill has felt much calmer, although her busy life is still very stressful.

The Dream Warrior

Rob was a 47-year-old chiropractor from California. He had been an oral surgeon and had also studied acupuncture, Oriental bodywork, reflexology, iridology, and Eastern philosophy. He was a black belt in martial arts and taught yoga classes. He had even prepared for a year to become a priest. Despite his busy practice, Rob meditated two hours a day. He described himself as "very goal-oriented and determined. My energy is normally very high, but I need a stimulus to get me going. I use herbal stimulants. I'm always having to know more, be more. I'm looking for total wholeness. I try to make people happy. I could easily give up my life for a cause or to save someone's life."

Rob was the life of the party and loved to do stand-up comedy acts. He enjoyed being at center stage. "I've read a lot about amazing people like Michelangelo, Buddha, and great comedians, and I have wondered what makes them tick. Great comedians have cynical minds. So do I. I have a cutting humor, but I'm not malicious. The other day I was in an elevator with an overweight woman. The back of her jeans said, "Guess." I said to myself, '500 pounds.' I make flippant, ridiculous jokes about people as I go through my day, then I make friends with them later. I make friends very easily."

Rob thrived on helping people. "I can see 80 to 90 patients a day, then feel more energized. It's a sympathetic adrenaline high. I have a tendency to overdo things. I'm good at everything I do. I never stop to pat myself on the back. My father always expected me to get 100 on every test. He'd criticize me if I got a 92 or a 95 and say nothing if I got 100. I was one of the top three table-tennis players in college. I'll do really well at something, then I'll leave it" Rob had a history of using lots of recreational drugs, especially during his long period of travel in South America.

What Rob wanted most was help with his irritability. It was the one underlying problem that he had not been able to shake. In high school, he had gotten into many fights. "There were always fights. I didn't want to get into them because of all the blood and teeth. But I knew I somehow had to protect myself and others. Whenever I get into an argument with someone, I tend to hang on to it. I'd really like to be able to let go of my anger." Rob's grandfather told him that he had noticed Rob always wanted to defend his point. Rob was embarrassed by his own anger. His father had a problem with anger, too.

There was something else very striking about Rob: his dreams. "My dreams have a continuous theme. I'm always fighting with someone, and I'm always the good guy, defending and helping people. I use hand-to-hand combat. Last week I had five dreams about fighting. I have them practically every night, sometimes several in one night. Most of the time I have to go correct something that's wrong. I wish these dreams would stop."

Rob also suffered from hemorrhoids and constipation. His joints popped too easily. He was very exercise-oriented and loved to run and work out. "I lose myself in it." He disliked being cold. Rob loved sweets and bread. He "would go wild with dairy," even though he should have avoided it because dairy caused him to suffer from sinus congestion.

Although Rob had not been diagnosed with ADHD, we recognized the impulsivity, daring quality, and his lack of follow through as typical characteristics of adults with ADHD. He would pick up an area of study or work, plunge into it wholeheartedly, then drop it and go on to something else. He was one of the most intense and fascinating people we had ever met. Rob had a superhuman aspect. What would normally take several people entire lifetimes to achieve, Rob accomplished in half his lifetime. Activities that would exhaust the average person gave him more energy. He exhibited a ceaseless yearning for the experiences of life and a tireless desire to help others. Rob demonstrated a type of hyperfocus that we often see in people with ADHD. Just as children become engrossed in Nintendo for hours on end, adults with ADHD can focus intensely on one thing, but move quickly from one task, or career, to another because of their need for constant stimulation and change. They need to have high levels of challenge in their waking hours, and sometimes even during their dreams.

We gave Rob one dose of *Agaricus muscaria,* a type of mushroom used as a hallucinogen by indigenous groups in various parts of the world. It is a medicine for people that undertake tremendous exploits and who also experience episodes of rage during which they are capable of great feats of strength. It is not surprising that Rob had actually used this mushroom many times while traveling in South America.

At his six-week follow-up visit, Rob told us, "I've never felt better. Before, I had dreams about conflict. I was always fighting with adversaries. I've only had these dreams a few times since taking the medicine. I haven't been irritable as much. My digestion is better."

Rob wrote us a letter five months later. "The medicine seems like the perfect match. I've had only two or three dreams of combat over the past five months. I used to have multiple combat dreams every single night. Gone! I hardly get angry anymore. I have more energy and I'm happier. I have more mental clarity, more focus, more purpose, and I feel closer to God. I'm also much less chilly. This is what you'd call a success story."

When we spoke with Rob by phone five months later, he reported, "I have lots of energy all the time. My dreams were fatiguing me. I always had to protect people. I'm talking about three, four, five battles a night. Sometimes I'd wake in the middle because my life was in danger, then I'd go back to sleep and renew the dream. I've had only three battle dreams since you gave me the medicine a year ago. Everything in my life has improved. I'm much more balanced and not as intense all the time. I'm more laid back, yet much more focused in general. My irritability has diminished tremendously. My hemorrhoids have only flared up a couple of times over the past year. I no longer have gas or bloating. Zero. My joints pop a lot less. I'm blossoming."

Rob has not needed another dose of *Agaricus* since the original dose.

I Live in a Constant State of Emergency

"I read an article about adult ADHD and it described me perfectly," Rebecca explained. "I'm kind of nervous. It's tough for me to wind down. I always have to be doing something, even if it's cleaning. I wish I could relax more. Since my son was born six years ago, I've felt like I was in a constant state of emergency. I've been rushing ever since. Other people can sit down and talk. Not me. I don't have the patience. They slow me down. Rushing, rushing, rushing. I just want to relax. It's no shock that I'm so crabby with all the hurrying."

"My acne rosacea started at the same time. They gave me antibiotics, which caused me to get a vaginal yeast infection. My hair began to gray when I was thirty."

"I keep to myself a lot. Probably because I get nervous around other people. It's hard for me to believe they're sincere. People talk about you behind your back, you know. When I get nervous, my mind freezes. I forget what I was talking about. Or I go into a room and can't remember why I went there. Doing so many things at one time makes it awfully hard to finish anything, which makes me even more impatient. I'm doing one thing and my mind is already on the next. Like imagining I'm out there doing all kinds of things while I'm actually in the shower. Since my son was born, I've never stopped rushing around."

"I grew up with this ADD. Never liked school so I used to skip classes and go to the library whenever I could. I still can't figure out how I ever passed or got the good grades that I did. As soon as I looked at a page of math, I got practically dizzy. What I remember most is not being able to think. I couldn't comprehend what I read unless it was something that genuinely interested me. My reports cards indicated that I had trouble listening and following directions since the first grade. I was never hyperactive, though."

It was in the fifth grade that I started getting mischievous, clowning around, and getting into trouble. Then, in junior-high school, I started skipping class. Don't remember bringing any work home half the time. The teachers kept saying I'd be a really good student if I only tried, but I never did. I pretty much wanted to avoid the whole school thing after junior-high school. I wasn't learning anything, was bored, and I didn't fit in. I got so far behind in math that I gave up on it. There were a few classes that I loved: business, typing, and American literature."

"My father was an alcoholic. Things would be normal for long periods, then he'd binge for a couple of days in a row and be crazy. We'd all be afraid to sleep. It went on till they divorced when I was a teenager. I got real wild around that time. Never seemed to worry about the consequences. I met a guy and moved in with him. He hit me a few times, and I tried to leave but didn't know where to go. I didn't want to cause trouble for anyone else. I don't know why I stayed. My boyfriend was so suspicious—watching me all the time. He finally went to jail, then life got better for me."

"As a kid, lightning and thunder scared me. I still hide when it's stormy outside. I don't like unprotected heights too much and snakes scare me, too. I get afraid they're gonna dart out at me, especially the big ones like rattlesnakes and copperheads. I'm afraid of horses, big dogs, and centipedes, too. And of skiing so fast that I can't stop. I would get so jumpy when my boyfriend walked into the room without my noticing that I would jump practically a mile high."

"I dream a lot, especially about flying or someone coming after me and killing me. When I was little, I had lots of snake dreams. I'd be walking down the road and a whole bunch of snakes would be on the path. It really happened once when I was a little girl. A big snake slithered right in front of me."

Rebecca felt different from other people, didn't like chitchat, and felt more comfortable sticking to herself. She worried that people didn't like her so she didn't even try to make friends. What if she made some stupid comment and then felt vulnerable? Her discomfort around others was exacerbated by her impatience with them.

We wondered if Rebecca's suspicious, keep-to-herself nature were triggered by her fear of her father's alcoholic rages. She had never connected the two, but admitted that she removed the light bulbs in her room during her father's binges so he couldn't see her and she could relax. She feared he'd beat her like he did her mother and once dreamed that he shot her from outside the bedroom window.

At the end of the interview, we inquired about Rebecca's tolerance of tight clothing. "I can't wait to remove my jeans," she replied. "I hated wearing turtlenecks as a kid and still do." We prescribed *Crotalus cascavella* (rattlesnake) for Rebecca based on her hurriedness, fear of being killed, aggravation from tight clothing, mistrust, her fears of snakes, centipedes, and horses, and of her dreams and contact with snakes. Even though Rebecca commented that she never was hyperactive with her ADD, the hurried tendency was present even as a child.

Rebecca responded dramatically to homeopathy. Not only did her acne rosacea and vaginitis clear up, but so did her mind. They improvement in the physical symptoms came first, then she no longer felt nervous around people. Rebecca felt calmer and, most importantly, her head cleared and her memory became much sharper. Her sexual energy returned after being gone for two years. Although some changes were immediate, it took five months for her to feel dramatically better and it has lasted. "I feel very different. Not so scattered. Much less frustrated with myself. Homeopathy has made such a difference in my life. It will always amaze me! When I read your book, it was one of those times when you just *know*—something is right. And it was." Rebecca's exuberant and bouncy son has also responded very positively to homeopathic treatment.

"I'm Scattered. It's Hard to Get on Track"

Genevieve, age forty, had never been formally diagnosed with ADHD, but many of her symptoms match the diagnostic criteria. She came to us primarily for her digestive problems, but also complained repeatedly about poor concentration. "I tend to forget things. I use lists or things do not get done. I don't work on a schedule. It's very hard to get on track. Life just doesn't flow easily. I understand the reasons why I'm so stressed, but I just can't handle them. There are so many demands, so many things for me to juggle. My husband and I misunderstand each other. We don't communicate well so there's friction.

"I'm scattered and have a hard time focusing. I have a good heart and my intentions are right, but there's so much going on. I'm constantly jumping from one thing to another. It's not new. It's the modus operandi that I've used for a long time. I like change, variety, people. But I'd like to be more centered instead of a feather in the wind or a butterfly. Before I had children, I used to just move whenever I felt like it. I must have lived in

seventeen different places in Arizona in just a couple of
years. Then I went back and forth to Central America.

"I really need harmony. I need to be in a better state
of balance, but I don't want to be a patient of anyone for
long. My track record of sticking with things isn't very
good. My husband's always telling me to finish what I
start. I feel like I'm failing in every area of my life and I
feel fragmented even talking about it. I'm not very good
at organizing things. In fact, I've bought so many orga-
nizers that I could open a second-hand store."

Genevieve had been diagnosed with diverticulosis
(the formation of pouches in the lining of the small intes-
tine), which caused her to feel bloated much of the time.
She came for help with her digestive problems and had
no idea that homeopathy could help her mind as well.

What we perceived as Genevieve's greatest limita-
tion was her mental fragmentation and her inability to
complete anything. She was indeed just like a feather
blowing in the wind, previously from home to home
and continent to continent, most recently from one
thought or idea to the next. We felt that the characteristics unique to Genevieve were: undertaking many
things, yet persevering and persisting in nothing and in-
constancy. We gave Genevieve *Plantago* (plantain).

People needing plant medicines are often plant-
like. Plants are sensitive, gentle, diffuse, changeable, and
move with the wind. This was definitely Genevieve's nature. Those needing *Plantago* can also be very confused,
so restless and nervous that they pace back and forth,
and do work hastily. The description "hurry or haste in
occupation; desire to do several things at once, but cannot finish anything" appears in the homeopathic literature under *Plantago* and certainly seems to depict
Genevieve perfectly. Genevieve returned five weeks later
to say that she felt much better. "The first thing that I no-

ticed was that I felt calmer, more patient. I was able to take a deep breath and be more still. I think I've found a centered place.

"I remember to write things down now. I'm clearer. I pick up more on details and am able to accomplish more. I'm not feeling as chaotic. I'm staying on track despite the fact that a lot of things have been going on. Although it's the nature of a mother to jump from one thing to another, I'm handling it better. I don't get frustrated as easily. My outbursts are really rare now. I used to get really upset over things I couldn't make go the way I wanted. My inner voice is talking louder and more clearly now."

The only time we had prescribed *Plantago* before was for dental pain, for which it had worked quite well. When Genevieve came for this first return visit, she mentioned that her teeth had been hurting quite a bit until she took the medicine. Now the pain was gone.

Homeopathic Treatment of Learning Disabilities, the Autism Spectrum, and Other Mental and Emotional Problems

18

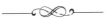

Enhancing the Learning Curve Through Homeopathy
Learning Disabilities and Developmental Delays

Approximately 800,000 children were classified as learning disabled in 1977. By 1986 this number had grown to 1.9 million. This is a different category from developmentally disabled children, whose numbers decreased over the same period of time by nearly 300,000, and the severely impaired group, which decreased by nearly 60,000. As of 1992, approximately 11 percent of all children enrolled in public schools received special education services.[1] As of 1996, 11.4 percent of children ages 6 to 21 were in special education, according to the U.S. Department of Education.[2] This percentage appears to be due to medical advances, increased diagnosis of ADHD and learning disabilities, the growing rate of social problems, and a desire among parents to place their disabled children with nondisabled students in public

---

[1] Sylvia Farnham-Diggory, *The Learning-Disabled Child* (Cambridge: Harvard University Press, 1992), 10, 12.

[2] Dana DiFilippo, Special Needs Multiplying, *The Cincinnati Enquirer,* September 26, 1999, <http://enquirer.com/editions/1999/09/26/loc_special_needs.html>.

schools.[3] We would add, from our clinical observation, a decreased tolerance among some teachers to have children with behavioral and learning disabilities in mainstream classrooms, as well as, in a positive light, greater awareness among parents and educators of the varied possibilities for individualized and special programs for children who are struggling.

In our practice, we treat many children who have an array of problems with concentration, information comprehension and retention, speech impairments and delays, and other communication problems. At the same time, a growing number of parents are seek alternative therapies for their children with problems on the autistic spectrum—most often autism, Asperger's disorder, pervasive developmental disorder, and a variety of more unusual genetic conditions, such as Down syndrome, Fragile X syndrome, Prader-Willi syndrome, and others.

This chapter includes both learning-disabled and severely impaired children, because we have found that children who are significantly developmentally delayed as well as children who are simply slow learners to benefit from homeopathic treatment. Our expectations as homeopathic physicians are, of course, different depending on the individual child. Children who are developmentally disabled, with or without behavioral problems, can sometimes achieve amazing strides in behavior, coping skills, and learning abilities. They continue to be substantially more limited in their capabilities than other children, unless the initial diagnosis was incorrect.

We have seen many children in learning-disabled school programs who are very bright. They may have poor self-confidence, inadequate learning styles, or a

---

[3] Ibid, p. 2.

family history of abuse or neglect, and received no encouragement to believe in themselves. They may be dyslexic, have auditory or visual problems, have no inspiring role models, suffer the physiologic consequences of their mothers' drug or alcohol abuse in utero, or simply be bored.

Each child has his own story to tell if we only take the time to listen. A youngster may need a different teacher, a new school, or may do much better learning at home. She may benefit from a radically different instructional approach designed to her individual learning style. Many of these children make tremendous strides after homeopathic treatment.

Dyslexia and Perfectionism

Kory, six years old, was a hands-on kind of kid. He loved cars, trucks, airplanes, Legos—anything mechanical. Energetic, bright, and inquisitive, Kory was "into his own thing." Although Kory seemed to get along pretty well with others, he was very sensitive to others referring to him as stupid or laughing at his mistakes. Group activities and team sports didn't appeal to him. Neither, unfortunately, did school. A kindergartner, Kory had an active and creative imagination, but his attention span was short. He had a hard time associating sounds with letters and had a habit of reversing or mistaking letters. He became even more confused if he was instructed what to write.

Difficult tasks frustrated Kory. He found it overly challenging to push beyond his limitations. A perfectionist, Kory would rather not do something if he couldn't do it well. Tests made him nervous, and he didn't like them. Any time Kory perceived that he did not do something well, he called it a failure and dwelled on his less-than-perfect achievements. "I messed up. It's all wrong," was a typical response. An unusually fastidious child, it really bothered Kory to get his hands dirty.

Crohn's disease (a potentially serious bowel condition characterized by abdominal cramping and diarrhea) ran on his mother's side of the family. Kory had his share of digestive problems, especially for a six-year-old. He suffered from frequent stomach pain, and diarrhea was an ongoing problem, in the form of "dumping" after every meal, and Kory's stools were very strong smelling. His anus tended to be raw during his episodes of loose bowel movements. Kory slept well but was slow to wake up in the morning.

China (Cinchona bark), which fits difficult concentration, periodic symptoms, stomach pain, and diarrhea took care of Kory's diarrhea completely, but there was no shift in his dyslexia. In fact, transposing letters and numbers and confusing left and right were his only remaining complaints.

The medicine that helped Kory with these remaining symptoms was *Germanium,* prescribed on the basis of his perfectionism, fear of failure, mistakes in writing and speaking, and dyslexia. Although this case is still in progress, over the past nine months two doses of *Germanium* have helped Kory's dyslexia, as well as his reading and his ability to differentiate left from right. He transposes letters much less often. Kory is not nearly as bothered that he doesn't do everything perfectly. His digestive problems never returned.

Naive, Gullible, and Literal

Justin was seven when his parents first contacted us. He had been diagnosed with Asperger's disorder, and

Justin's parents were especially concerned about his limited abilities to function appropriately around others. "He's in his own world," his mother began. "Sometimes he can't even carry on a two-way conversation. Or he'll chime in with a comment that's completely irrelevant." A late talker, Justin's vocabulary was limited to twenty words until he was four years old. Justin often acted without any apparent awareness. Naive, gullible, literal—all of these describe Justin well. Justin's attention was very limited and his distractibility had caused the school to bring pressure to bear on his parents. This child caught on quickly to simple concepts, but definitely needed a structured environment to learn.

Justin was always different from the other kids—singing to himself, distracted, oblivious to social cues. He didn't look at people directly and talked when others weren't even listening to him. His conversation was often repetitive, and he could perseverate on the tiniest details of his computer games. During the interview, Justin continued to elaborate on the intricacies of Nintendo and Winnie-the-Pooh. Justin was a clumsy child and hadn't a clue about playing soccer. He loved splashing around in the pool during the summer, but had never actually learned to swim. He also loved to play with his Beanie Babies.

A mover, Justin paced three steps, turned, then paced again. This child had a very loud voice and was prone to screaming. When in an impulsive, out-of-control mood, Justin fingered anything around him and, when really upset, threatened, "I'm gonna kill her!" but it was obvious that his words were empty. He was also known to jump on or fight with his brother, Lyndon, and had wrapped a radio cord around Lyndon's neck. Despite his aggressive tendencies, he was a helpful boy who loved his family. This youngster would do anything to get attention from adults. When his parents talked to each other, Justin did whatever he could to get them to stop and do what he wanted instead.

We asked Justin's mom about her pregnancy with him. It turned out that she and Justin's father had suffered a great deal of discord and that she feared he might abandon her as a previous boyfriend had done. Upon probing more deeply, we discovered that Justin's mother had felt that she was not good enough, that no matter how she behaved, someone would eventually leave her.

Justin's physical complaints included "an itchy butt," a tendency towards loose stools, and a prolonged outbreak of hives for nine months after receiving his MMR (measles, mumps, and rubella) immunization. Another homeopath had treated Justin with *Sulphur*, which produced a partial improvement.

The only homeopathic medicine that Justin has needed is *Baryta sulphuricum* (barium sulphate). Barium covers Justin's shyness, delayed development, and awkwardness. *Sulphur* is an excellent match for the tendency to be in his own world, obliviousness to social cues, and his mother's feeling of being scorned which, we believe, could have affected Justin.

After two-and-a-half months, Justin's mom described her son as more aware and less in his own world. His spelling had improved, he was not as wild or unruly, was able to socialize more, and appeared to be developing a sense of empathy. These positive changes continued over the following months; his temper flared less often, he no longer hurt others, and he made violent, if empty, threats less frequently. The pacing and circling stopped, and he became more adept at two-way conversations. It has been a year and four months since Justin began homeopathic treatment, and he has needed

Baryta sulphuricum six times. He has not needed any psychiatric medications, and his parents rave about their new and improved child.

Autistic and Electric

Tyler's mother first consulted with us by telephone in the fall of 1997 from Ottawa. As with many of our patients, we have never met Tyler personally. His diagnosis was autism and his mother, after reading *Ritalin-Free Kids*, wondered if homeopathy might help Tyler, who was by now ten years old. "It wasn't a bad pregnancy," she told us, "just a lot of tiredness and morning sickness." Then the excitement began. Tyler was two weeks overdue, his mother's water broke, and they suffered the first blizzard of the season. Only one obstetrician was on call for two hospitals, and he was already busy with a delivery at the other hospital. Tyler's pulse became weak. The doctor was involved in an auto accident on his way to the hospital. Five hours later, Tyler was born by Caesarean section!

Tyler's mom noticed that he was rather flaccid compared to other babies. Unable to settle down, he slept poorly. His mom quit breast feeding at three months and went back to work when he was six months old, at which time he was placed in day care. Tyler experienced numerous episodes of otitis media and conjunctivitis, as well as a couple of bouts of bronchitis.

Tyler's parents always felt there was something different about him. Though quite precocious when it came to objects, their baby was not much interested in people. He was fascinated with light switches and buttons. By the age of two years, his development appeared to be regressing rather than progressing. He spoke only one word at a time, usually to express some sort of demand, then continued to scream until his object of desire was put in his hand. Demanding and restless, he insisted on being held and accompanied around the house and refused to stay in his crib.

Taking Tyler anywhere, in the words of his mom, "was a nightmare." He'd bolt across six aisles at the supermarket at the blink of an eye. His poor mom needed to be on alert every minute of every day. Tyler delighted in stuffing objects into electric sockets and was able to remove the safety plugs even faster than his mother. He loved to hide things, and, particularly, to put them down the heating vents. His mother still had not located some of the pieces of jewelry that he had hidden. Tyler slept only four to six hours a night and never napped from the age of twelve months. His weary parents slept even less!

The family moved to a different province when Tyler was three and a half. He went wild; his behavior became even more erratic. When he entered a second day care six months later, his behavior was totally different from that of any of the other children. Tyler isolated himself and preferred to play alone. At this point, a psychiatrist misdiagnosed him with attention deficit/hyperactivity disorder, a diagnosis that, unfortunately, stuck with him for four years. Tyler's vocabulary did not develop, and it was impossible to get his attention. His parents wondered if he were deaf. Unable to recognize letters or colors, he would not participate in school projects and was very slow to learn anything. In addition, Tyler had the habit of walking on his tiptoes.

Tyler's behavior began to deteriorate. He hit, bit, and slapped his classmates and was unwilling to cooperate with his teacher. A psychiatrist prescribed Ritalin, which resulted in some behavioral improvement.

It was at this point that Tyler's mother consulted us. He was now in a regular classroom but was categorized learning disabled in some subjects. Tyler's teachers observed him to be very anxious about trying to keep up with the other children. Any little thing would set him off, provoking him to cry, scream, lose his temper, and pace about hysterically. When frustrated, he could squeeze his dog too tightly. He had a habit of insisting things were a certain way even if he was obviously wrong. The psychiatrist added Dexedrine to the Ritalin.

Without his medications, Tyler was very antsy and walked around in circles. He'd flick his pencil, fidget with the glue bottle, and wander around the classroom talking to himself. Not only did he not seek out other children on the playing field, but he also didn't even seem to see them. He refused to interact with the other children unless forced to do so and turned his back on adults who wanted to assist him. Although Tyler had good reasoning skills and was sharp with equations and complicated games, body language went right over his head. He was unable to generalize his learning and to readily switch from one activity to the next.

Tyler had several other quirks. When tiny, he hated water and still didn't appreciate getting his face wet. Haircuts and combing were painful events for Tyler. He loved to do mischievous things like pour shampoo down the drain or sprinkle powder all over the bathroom to create what his mother called "a winter wonderland." With quite a mechanical bent, once he even figured out how to stop the luggage carousel at the airport. When flashlight batteries disappeared, Tyler's parents knew he was the culprit. He also walked in his sleep and suffered from nightmares; previously he had had inconsolable night terrors. Tyler, however, was quite fearless and thought nothing of walking to the edge of a cliff while his terrified parents held their breath.

It was no problem identifying unique traits in this young man. Although his tendency to isolate, pace, difficulty switching gears, combination of precocity and learning disability, and even his tiptoeing, are fairly common to autistic children, many of his other symptoms were odd. These included his fascination with electric sockets and other mechanical devices; his fear of water, night terrors, and tendency to bite; and his somnambulism. Tyler was no ordinary child.

Tyler benefited considerably from homeopathic *Helium,* a medicine for children who are nonreactive, unapproachable, and distant. It is curious that helium, as a substance, possesses no electrical resistance and, therefore, climbs up the walls of containers as if to defy gravity. Just like Tyler when he fearlessly approached steep precipices.

Within two months, Tyler's mother noticed some impressive changes. More attentive to making friends, he also began to experience increasingly adventurous dreams about conversing with other people. His walking around in circles diminished, and he was much less sensitive to being teased. Tyler began to narrate information to his parents in the most minute detail. He was now able to break away from a conversation appropriately and move on to the next task. Tyler was able to comb his own hair without pain. The sleepwalking ceased, and he was gentler in his interactions with the family's dog.

We did not hear from Tyler's mother again until almost six months later. She had felt he was doing quite well. In cases of children with significant developmental problems, we have found that it is often better to allow several months to elapse between visits in order to evaluate the full extent of progress. Now Tyler was more keyed into playing with other children. There was still no more sleepwalking, and his impulsivity remained better. His verbal skills had improved.

Over the following year, Tyler continued to show gains on all levels, both at home and at school. More adaptable to life in general, his frustration level was much lower and his dietary repertoire was much expanded. He no longer found twenty different excuses to avoid doing whatever was asked of him. His mother rated impulsivity as "almost 100 percent better." Pushing buttons and snarling up the television controls were no longer an issue. Tyler was still in a learning-disabilities class for reading and writing, but was steadily improving. In fact, he was on the honor roll at the end of the year. The teachers commented that his scores would be admirable for any child. He was able to pick up most of his classmates' names. If a topic interested Tyler, he was quite verbal. He even made it through haircuts at the barbershop without screaming.

Tyler's parents had chosen to keep him on his medications despite his improvement with homeopathy. After a year, however, they realized that it no longer made any difference when he forgot to take his Dexedrine. This was the first time that Tyler had, of his own initiative, asked to talk to us. He chatted about being moved to a mainstream classroom and shared that it no longer bothered him much if other kids picked on him. His mother reported that Tyler needed less assistance in the classroom, was better handling his responsibilities, and turning in his assignments promptly. At that point, it was possible to taper off the Dexedrine.

Two years after we first treated him, the complaints weren't nearly as extreme as earlier. *Helium* had helped

Tyler considerably, but his main problem was vegetating on the couch after school, being more involved with his Power Rangers than with those around him, and being disinterested in bathing. We gave him one dose of *Sulphur*, which allowed him to interact more with his peers, to be less in his own world, and to complete his assignments. The *Sulphur* was repeated six months later when he began to relapse, after which his symptoms again improved. Usually we find that a single homeopathic medicine repeated at infrequent intervals is most effective. Tyler, however, benefited from three medicines: *Helium, Sulphur,* and, most recently, *Helleborus* (black hellebore), which has allowed him to take a further step toward appropriate social interaction. His mother currently estimates a 75 to 80 percent improvement as a result of homeopathic treatment.

The Boy Who Could Not Stop Kissing

Jerry, a seventeen year old with a significant developmental disability, was tall, blond, well built, and had a very sweet, childlike expression and affect. He smiled most of the time. We noticed, on his first visit five-and-a-half years ago, that he had no eyebrows. His mother explained that he had just shaved them off. Jerry crawled and sat at nine months and walked at two-and-a-half years. At the age of three he was diagnosed with mid-range mental retardation and an IQ of 50. The cause did not seem to be genetic.

As long as his mother could remember, Jerry had problems with coordination and depth perception. He suffered from seizures from ages three to thirteen, for which he received anticonvulsant medications. Jerry had a very short attention span and was unable to maintain eye contact. His hands were always busy, and he was always grabbing one thing or another. From infancy he only took five-minute naps, and slept five to six hours a night. By age ten Jerry was so hyperactive that his mother could not find a babysitter who could cope with his activity level.

Jerry was in a special-education high school where he would receive career training and job placement. He could only sit still for one hour at a time. Generally happy all the time, he loved to tease others. He grabbed people's wrists and liked to hug and kiss them. He even hugged and kissed inanimate objects like escalator rails and trucks. He was still uncoordinated. He had recently dived into a swimming pool for the first time.

Although Jerry had a delightful, playful temperament, others often found him overwhelming and playfully aggressive. His teachers reported that he picked on weak kids and harassed them. He enjoyed being the center of attention. He played with light switches and fire alarms.

Very limited verbally, Jerry often communicated through pantomime. His verbal skills were limited to "mama," "dada," "truck," and other simple, monosyllabic words. He was unable to enunciate clearly, so most of his words sounded the same. He easily forgot whatever he learned.

Jerry's judgment was poor. If his mother did not watch him closely, he would wander off. He did so a year before we met him and was hit by a car, resulting in two fractures of the left foot. He would use half a roll of toilet paper or none at all. If left alone, he did mischievous things like putting antifreeze in the crankcase.

He was shy when meeting new people. As a child he would walk around with a towel over his head if there were guests. Jerry loved animals but did not know how to be gentle with them. He picked up cats by the neck, though he never meant to hurt them. He rarely showed anger and was afraid of his stepfather's temper. He never cried much. Jerry needed lots of reassurance.

He had very few physical complaints, just some facial acne and a tendency to stiff joints. Jerry loved sweets.

Many of Jerry's characteristics are very typical of developmentally disabled people. Homeopathy always looks for what is unique and atypical about an individual. Jerry's constant busyness and his impulse to hug and kiss everyone were outstanding to us. We prescribed *Veratrum album* for Jerry. People needing this medicine, in addition to being constantly busy and hurried as mentioned previously, can have the specific symptom of wanting to touch and kiss everything. Jill, mentioned earlier, was an adult with a high degree of impulse control and was able to restrain herself from acting on her impulses in order to be socially acceptable. Jerry, who was unable to control his impulses, kissed with abandon.

As with many of the other patients we have presented, Jerry took only one dose of the *Veratrum*. His mother brought him back to our office four months later. She reported that he acted out more for a while after taking the medicine, then his behavior improved dramatically. He no longer kissed inappropriately. His attention span was longer, his eye contact improved, and his judgment was better. He had recently spent a whole day moving a woodpile, which he never would have been able to do before. His listening had gotten a lot better and so had his coordination. Jerry noticed recently that he was dropping something and caught it before it hit the floor, which was extremely unusual for him. His reactions were quicker now and he was better able to catch balls. Before the homeopathy, he would throw the ball up on the roof and start laughing. Now he threw and caught it very well. He also kicked the ball appropriately, which was a new behavior. He enjoyed playing with the ball so much that he wanted to do it all day.

Jerry was attending better to tasks. He was putting away all of his clothes instead of stopping in the middle. The teachers reported that he was much better about refraining from touching others. The day camp counselor said that his behavior had improved greatly over the previous year. Jerry's mother noticed that he was trying to talk more. He had begun to sing in front of others, even the whole neighborhood. He was now trying to put endings on words. He retained information better and his enunciation had even improved a bit. He had taken cooking classes for years, but only since the medicine did he start to prepare his mother's breakfast. He could now make French toast appropriately, although he still needed help to turn the burner to the right temperature. Jerry has needed only five repetitions of the *Veratrum* over the past five and a half years.

It Took Todd Two Hours to Decide Which Toy He Wanted

Todd had bright red hair, a full face, red cheeks, and was considerably overweight for a nine-year-old. He was developmentally delayed and in a special-education class. His mother was also developmentally disabled. Todd's father was unknown. He had an older brother of normal intelligence and a developmentally delayed sister three years older who had the habit of biting and clawing Todd. He compensated by eating. Todd, who was now living with his mother's sister, had gone from 63 to 104 pounds in five months.

Todd was not good at participating in group activities with his peers. He took balls and toys away from other children and ignored them when they objected. He disregarded reprimands of all kinds. He was very restless. His aunt did not like to take him to the store because he wandered off. He was too friendly with strangers.

Todd had great difficulty making decisions. If his aunt took him to the toy store, it took him two hours to decide what he wanted. He sometimes became violent without apparent provocation. Two weeks before we first saw him, he slapped and hit the school bus driver. He frequently misunderstood what was said to him and sat unresponsively, not knowing what to do or how to follow instructions. His learning abilities were extremely impaired because he often seemed to have no idea what the teacher expected of him. Todd was unable to read.

Todd did not masturbate, but he would strip down, naked, in front of others. He did not care about his appearance and often walked around with several inches of his bottom exposed. He scratched his genitals in public without any embarrassment.

Todd's chief physical complaint was a micropenis. His genitals were not fully formed at birth. He had been treated with testosterone injections at ages three and four without success. It was hard for him to stand and urinate because his penis was too small to hold comfortably, though the urine came out adequately. His testicles were also small since birth, and he had surgery for undescended testicles at age three. Todd had an obvious speech impediment, particularly when he pronounced the letter *S*. His cheeks flushed easily, and he did not have much stamina. He preferred to take elevators rather than walk up stairs. His feet got hot easily.

Todd's main psychological and behavioral problems were his apparent lack of intelligence, inability to grasp basic instructions, and lack of awareness of his impact on others. We originally gave Todd a dose of *Baryta carbonica* (barium carbonate) with no effect. When a medicine is given that does not best match the symptoms of the individual, there is usually no response whatsoever.

After restudying Todd's case, we realized that what was most unusual about Todd was the combination of his limited intellectual capabilities and his shamelessness about being naked in public. We prescribed *Bufo* (toad), a homeopathic medicine often prescribed for children with significant delay or limitations in learning, who may be much brighter than they appear. They seem dull and are often unable to grasp complex or sophisticated concepts. They may not function at grade level, but may be highly capable at one isolated skill or talent, like an idiot savant. They may appear stupid physically, sometimes with a protruding tongue. Often people

Bufo rana (toad)

The poisonous sweat from a toad is used in homeopathy as a medicine for slow, coarse children with a particularly strong interest in sex and masturbation. These children do not comprehend very well. They often have a dull look on their faces as well as thick lips, which they lap with their tongue. They rely mainly on basic instincts and instant gratification. Music or bright objects are intolerable to them. They have a particular aversion to being misunderstood. Seizures are common.

needing *Bufo* have a shameless or inordinate fixation on sex and a propensity to frequent masturbation. The character James in the movie *To Die For* fits *Bufo* well. The young man was slow-witted and spent his evenings masturbating in front of porno videos. He was willing to do absolutely anything, even commit murder, to gratify himself sexually. Even when sentenced to life in prison, his sexual encounters continued in the form of dreams.

Two months after Todd took *Bufo,* his aunt called to say he was no longer having problems holding his penis during urination. His penis appeared to be an inch longer within six weeks after the medicine. He had also lost a significant amount of weight. Todd's aunt took him to a urologist who confirmed the increase in penis size and told her it could not be fully explained by the weight loss. Todd's cheeks were no longer flushed. We last heard about Todd one year later. He had transferred into a regular first grade classroom and continued to do very well.

He's Off in His Own World

Shakur, five years old, sang and talked normally until he was two, at which time his mother used drugs, moved out of the house temporarily, and left him with his grandmother. Shakur's mother used cocaine, drank beer, and smoked cigarettes throughout the pregnancy. He was born after six months in utero and weighed one pound thirteen ounces. He suffered from chronic lung disease since birth and needed a respirator for the first three years of his life. Afterward he had taken a number of asthma medications. Even now, when he developed a severe cold, Shakur was put on a respirator to facilitate his breathing and prevent asthma. He was found to have a congenital heart murmur at two months of age and was hospitalized for nine months at that time.

We noticed that Shakur grimaced and made unintelligible sounds throughout the interview. One striking thing about this child was that he looked just like a little old man. His grandmother described him as very hyperactive with a short attention span. He moved all the time. Unable to communicate verbally, he was off in his own world whether or not other children were around. He preferred playing by himself and seemed unable to connect with other children. Shakur clapped his hands loudly, even in the middle of the night. When frustrated, he clapped even more violently. The clapping stopped shortly after his mother returned from a drug treatment center. He frequently jerked his head from side to side and sometimes jerked his whole upper torso convulsively. He made lots of spastic motions and gestures. The child shrieked loudly and cried fearfully whenever he was around a Nintendo game.

Shakur often screamed to get his mother's attention. He said "Hi" to his mother in the morning and stroked her face. Occasionally he even greeted her with "G'morning." The more excited he became, the more sounds he made. He was unable to control his behavior in an open area because he was all over the place. He frequently growled. He liked to roll in the dirt or grass or on thick carpets like a little puppy dog. He put his mouth on everything and loved to lick things. He liked loud noises like drums. Pain did not seem to bother Shakur; he never cried when he hurt himself. Shakur hated doctors and examinations.

Shakur's grandmother had no idea if homeopathic treatment could help him, but she knew another family we had treated and wanted to give it a try. She told us it

Zincum metallicum (zinc)

Children corresponding to the picture of this medicine are fidgety and restless; their nervous system is overamped, with twitching, jerking, and even convulsions. The keynote symptom for this medicine is restless legs in bed. They complain a lot. They are sensitive, irritable, and can go into rages. With a persistent feeling of having committed a crime, they worry about being chased by the police. Their minds can be dull, with mistakes in speaking and writing. These children sometimes have a tendency to lick everything. They can look like little old people.

was as if Shakur were stuck somewhere and she wanted to help him find his way out.

There were many aspects of Shakur's behavior and personality that were unique. He had come into the world as a crack baby, and the genetic odds were not in his favor. Due to his low birth weight and premature birth, Shakur's lungs were not fully developed and continued to show weakness. His heart murmur indicated an inherent cardiovascular debility. In cases such as Shakur's, the homeopath does not expect a full recovery but a definite improvement. The extent of the improvement is up to the individual. Shakur's constant motion was notable, especially the spastic, jerking quality. So was his propensity for licking everything. His autistic-like tendencies, high pain threshold, and animal-like behaviors were also striking. The one word that sums up Shakur's state is convulsive. His every action, gesture, and word was expressed in a jerk or a spasm.

For this reason, we prescribed for him *Zincum metallicum* (zinc). It is an important homeopathic medicine for spastic, jerking, convulsive motions, and hyper-activity. People needing this medicine tend to have two unusual characteristics that we found in Shakur: the appearance of an old man and an impulse to lick objects, both animate and inanimate.

Shakur's grandmother did not bring him back to see us for four months. At that time she reported, and we readily noticed, that he had calmed down tremendously. He had begun to enunciate some words including "Momma" and even phrases like "What's up, daddy?" His teacher noticed that his attention span was longer.

Shakur could play with toys now. He had begun to interact with other children and was in his own world only 40 percent of the time now instead of 100 percent. He still screamed and licked everything. He had started to cry when in pain. Shakur still growled like an animal. He was no longer jerking his head, though he still exhibited some spastic motions. Even we were astounded by how much Shakur had changed.

During the ten months that we treated Shakur, he continued to improve. He stopped licking objects, was able to concentrate on watching cartoons for brief periods of time, and learned to play tag and basketball. His screaming diminished and his head jerking occurred only when he danced to rhythmic music. His vocabulary was still minimal. At this point we moved our office twenty minutes north of Seattle, and Shakur's grandmother no longer brought him to see us despite our offer of continuing to treat him by telephone. We were very sad that he could no longer receive homeopathic treatment because he seemed to benefit dramatically. We are often asked if homeopathy can help crack babies and children born with fetal alcohol syndrome. Shakur's case gives us a glimpse of the possibilities of homeopathy with such challenged children.

19

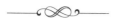

A Terrifying World
Fearful, Anxious Kids

Homeopathy: An Answer for Many a Frightened Child

It is rare that we meet a child who does not admit to some kind of fear. Or, even if the child is determined to look cool and insists he is free of fears, the parent will usually acknowledge that the child has one or more fears or phobias. Take, for example, a 21-year-old wrestler whom we recently interviewed. The kid was tough to the max. His only desire in life was to pin down his opponents. The bigger they were, the greater the challenge. Infuriated when he got into a fight and his friends didn't defend him, this young man appeared to be absolutely fearless. Only at the end of several interviews did he happen to mention his lifelong fear of receiving injections or having blood drawn.

Fears sometimes arise after traumatic events such as the death of a parent, abandonment, physical or sexual abuse, family violence, or an attack by an animal. But the causative factor or event can be more subtle, ongoing, or insidious, such as witnessing ongoing verbal abuse between parents or years of frightening, violent acts in television, movies, video games, or computer games.

Child psychology books attribute certain fears to particular ages of children. For example, from birth to six months, children are said to fear loud noises and lack of support. Fear of separation is said to come later, when the child is one to two years old. Two-year-olds are said to develop fears of imaginary creatures, burglars, and large approaching objects. At three, psychologists explain, children develop fears of animals, the dark, and being alone. Four-year-old youngsters are said to fear loud noises, such as fire engines, the dark, wild animals, and their parents' leaving at night. At five, more concrete fears arise, such as injury, falling, and dogs. At age six, they talk of fears of ghosts, witches, and someone under the bed as well as of natural disasters. More sophisticated fears arise from ages seven to ten, such as fears of failure and criticism, death, the unknown, and medical and dental procedures.[4] Experts even go so far as to quantify the number of fears children experience. One study concluded that children ages two to six have an average of three fears and that 40 percent of children ages six to twelve have as many as seven fears.[5] We wonder how adults would score!

This list and numerical assessment of fears are interesting, but homeopaths emphasize each child's individual experience and select a corresponding medicine. If you ask your child to describe her fears or nightmares, you may be surprised at the candid response. During our interviews over the years, children have often revealed to us, in the presence of their parents, fears about which their parents had not a clue. A child's fears, whether or not the parent may find them logical or believable, can provide considerable insight into that

[4] Schroeder and Gordon, op. cit., 315.
[5] Ibid., 323.

child's state. Homeopathy can often alleviate fears and phobias, regardless of their origins. Whether the specific fear revolves around attending school, separating from parents, monsters, wild animals, germs, thunderstorms, bridges, dying, snakes, or impending danger, a homeopathic medicine usually corresponds to the state of the child as a whole, which can also help diminish the fears significantly.

Fears can remain with people even as adults. One thirty-eight-year-old patient with ADHD told us that she has been afraid of the dark ever since childhood and still is today. As a little girl, she ran as fast as she could from light switch to light switch to avoid the terrifying blackness. In her twenties she lay in bed at night frightened that evil spirits might surround her in the darkened room. Now she still finds the dark scary but, as a parent trying to help her child cope with her own fears, has learned to handle her own.

A Matter of Life and Death

Annie, six years old, had always demanded to sleep in her parents' bed. She slept well for the first two-and-a-half months of her life and was a good nurser. After that, her mom could no longer produce enough milk and put Annie on formula. She woke several times a night until she reached the age of five. She still wanted to sleep with her parents. Her mother tried to put her to sleep in her own bed. Annie told her she was afraid and would not go to sleep unless her mother lay down next to her until she fell asleep. Otherwise she would lie in bed and cry. She always woke up during the night and went into her parents' bed.

Annie's mom described her as high-strung and tense. Even as a baby, she was like a little adult in a child's body. As she grew, Annie was quite bright, quick to catch on to anything new. She thought more like an adult than a child. Annie had a controlling personality and had the habit of dictating instructions to her parents as if she were the adult and they were the kids. She expected them to do just as they were told.

Annie's parents had been married for twenty-five years. She was very attached to her twenty-three-year-old sister and wanted her sister and her mom at home with her at all times. Even when she went over to her sister's house she called her mother again and again. This little girl did not even want her mother to go to the neighborhood store without taking her along.

Annie's fear of being alone began four months earlier. The whole family contracted food poisoning, but Annie's case was the worst. She had experienced severe stomach cramps and vomiting. Ever since that time, she was panicky that she would get food poisoning again. She insisted that she could not go to school because her stomach might hurt (this was before her homeschooling began).

Annie's fear about her health became so severe that she hated to leave her house and did not even want her parents to go out. She became frightened of going out in the car even with her mother there. She tried to jump out of the car twice because she wanted to go home. Sometimes, when Annie's mom went out and left her at home with her older sister, she had to rush back home because Annie would call her to say she was doubled over with abdominal pain. As soon as she knew her mother was on her way home, she felt fine. Whenever her mother tried to leave without her, Annie would become hysterical and claw at her mother in an attempt to hang on to her and prevent her from going anywhere. Lately Annie cried the whole time her mother was gone. She refused to go to school, so her mother decided to homeschool her.

Annie's mother had experienced considerable emotional distress during her pregnancy. She had an older son at the time and, during the first few months of the pregnancy, felt trapped and afraid of having another child whose demands she needed to meet. She cried a lot during that time. The rest of the pregnancy went very well. Annie was delivered by Caesarean section because of her sideways presentation in the birth canal. She was put in a neonatal ward for nine hours after her birth due to respiratory problems. From the time her mother stopped nursing, Annie became restless. She continued to want a bottle "forever" (until she was four years old).

Annie was a skillfully demanding child who nagged until she got her way. She always worried about when things were going to happen. Annie counted down the days before any event that she awaited.

She was extremely sloppy. Her room looked like a bomb struck five minutes after she cleaned it. Annie's mother had gone back to work full-time when Annie was four months old. Annie would be mad at her mother when she came home and clearly resented her for not being there. She had never been in a daycare situation. Recently Annie was very afraid of people breaking into her house. On a family vacation to Hawaii, some people appeared to be casing their condominium. This terrified Annie.

She developed occasional fevers up to 101 degrees Fahrenheit, at which time she became delirious and saw witches with long nails. She was a very restless sleeper. She loved pizza, spaghetti, candy, nachos, and chocolate milk.

And so, the homeopath wonders, what is most unusual about Annie? Her fear of robbers? No. Anyone who had the experience Annie's family had in Hawaii might develop some apprehension about their house being robbed. Her sloppiness? No, this is fairly typical of children Annie's age.

We felt that what was most outstanding about Annie was her desperate fear of being alone and her exaggerated possessiveness of her mother arising from this terror. It was as if Annie would die if her needs weren't met immediately. Annie's life was extremely limited by her belief that she would be in danger if her mother was not in her immediate proximity to protect her. This fear prevented her from feeling comfortable going to school or even spending the night at a friend's house.

We first saw Annie two-and-a-half years ago. She has benefited a great deal from the homeopathic medicine *Arsenicum album,* derived from arsenic. People needing this medicine are anxious, fearful, and nervous. They are afraid that others are going to rob them, and they have a deep insecurity about their safety and their ability to survive in the world. Individuals sometimes need this medicine if one of their parents has died or abandoned them, or even if they merely perceive abandonment, such as when Annie's mother went back to work. It is possible in Annie's case that this perceived aloneness in the world and fundamental feeling of danger and insecurity began in her first hours of life when she was taken away from her mother for nine hours because of her respiratory distress. This is not to say that Annie's mother should have done anything differently, but to show how early in life these beliefs and impressions can arise.

Five weeks after beginning homeopathic treatment, Annie's mother brought her back to see us and reported

Arsenicum album (arsenic)

Restless and insecure, children fitting the picture of *Arsenicum* have a lot of anxiety about their health and often fear death, as someone feels who has been poisoned with arsenic. They can also exhibit great concern about germs and contamination and a disproportionate terror of being left alone. These children are more anxious and adult-like than a child should be at his or her age. They are needy, whiny, and impatient. Burning pains, asthma, diarrhea, and stomachaches are common in these children. Often freezing, they like the warmth of a stove, fire, or their favorite blankie. When thirsty, they often prefer to sip liquids throughout the day.

that she was much less clingy. Now she was able to stay with her older sister or with a baby-sitter. Her mother still called to check in every so often. Annie's mother now revealed that her daughter used to call for her even when she needed to go to the bathroom. When her mother answered, Annie would reply, "Just checking." Not anymore. She still wanted her mother to be present when she went to bed, but was now able to sleep next to her parents' bed instead of in it. She now slept through the night rather than waking up and crawling into bed with her mother. Annie would now go to the bathroom and for a drink of water alone at church, which had been impossible for her previously. She still preferred to be homeschooled, to which her mother agreed.

Annie went through another phase of being very afraid she would get sick. She became worried about germs and insisted that her mother boil the family water.

This overconcern about health and germs is also common in people needing *Arsenicum*.

Two years later, Annie was doing much better. She no longer worried about getting sick and completely forgot about needing to drink boiled water. People did not make her feel nervous anymore. Annie's mother described her as much less high-strung and excitable. She felt fine in elevators and on bridges, which had made her uncomfortable in the past. Her mother told us that she had never remembered to tell us that Annie's concentration was also much improved after homeopathy. She also mentioned that Annie used to tackle her little nephew and even hit and punched him when she was upset. She now treated him much more gently.

Holding on to Mom for Dear Life

At age four, Hayley was a very sweet little girl with beautiful platinum hair and blue eyes. She came from a very loving, tight-knit family of six. Her mother homeschooled all of the children. Hayley was "mommy's girl." Like Annie, Hayley was very clingy and cried for her mom to be with her. She usually slept through the night in a bed with an older sister, but still crawled into her parents' bed in the middle of the night about twice a week. Hayley insisted on lying across her mother's lap all the time, even as she slept, her arms entwined around her mother's legs. Hayley clung tightly to her mother or her sister. When the family went to church on Sunday, Hayley refused to go to the nursery with the other children, insisting instead on staying with her mom.

Hayley loved looking pretty and wearing her favorite dresses, especially if they were frilly and lacy. Quick to cry when upset or whenever she got hurt, she made a mad dash for her mother, the only one capable of comforting her. A chatterbox, she was forever filled with burning questions. She expressed great frustration when she did not think others were listening to her or they tried to finish her sentences for her. Hayley thrived on telling other people what to do, regardless of their age.

If her mom were around, Hayley demanded that she do every little thing for her. Otherwise she could be quite independent. She usually behaved very well, but when she did not, everyone in the house knew that she was unhappy. A fussy infant, Hayley had accustomed her mom to carrying her around to calm her, much more so than with her three siblings. It seemed to her mom that all she did for the first year or two of Hayley's life was to hold and satisfy her little bundle of joy. She nursed until the age of two.

Hayley was quite healthy except for a history of recurrent middle ear infections resulting in surgery to implant ear tubes at the age of eighteen months. The only problem she had since was a thick nasal discharge when she got a cold. At these times she wanted, as always, to be on her mom's lap. Her mother, who had read about homeopathic acute prescribing, had given her *Pulsatilla* (windflower) several times for these colds with good results. Hayley had been difficult to potty train and still wet the bed sometimes. She loved to take off her shoes and socks and to kick off the covers at night. She loved to have cold air blowing on her. Hayley liked ice cream, cheese, and peanut butter and jelly and had an average level of thirst.

Distinguishing between Annie's and Hayley's cases will give you a good idea of how a homeopath makes fine distinctions among children. Annie and Hayley were both very dependent on their mothers and both wanted to be with their mothers all of the time, even in bed at night. But the two little girls' natures were different in other ways. Annie had a more intense and desperate nature. Her preoccupations went beyond fear of being alone without her mother and extended to fear of germs and robbers. She could strike out at her nephew when angry. Hayley had a sweeter, gentler disposition. Her only problem was her excessive clinginess. Hayley reminded us of yet another child whose mother described her daughter as "the Velcro kid," because she always wanted to be stuck to her mom. It was not even enough for Hayley to sit or lay on her mother's lap; she had to be wrapped around her. Loving as her mother was, it got to be just too much closeness. Hayley's dad, who had cut the umbilical cord of her three older siblings, joked that the doctor who cut hers just did not have the knack.

The first medicine that we prescribed for Hayley, *Pulsatilla*, had only a partial effect on her clinginess. The typical response to a medicine that is not the best match for a person is only slight or none at all. We restudied Hayley's case and prescribed for her a less common medicine, one known for its extreme clinginess. In fact the

Bismuthum subnitucum (bismuth)

This medicine is well suited to children who cling desperately to their parent's hand out of terror of being alone. They even follow the parent to the bathroom out of fear of being alone for a few minutes. We have heard these children called "Velcro kids." Solitude is unbearable. Bismuth is helpful for acute stomach pain in which even water is vomited as soon as it reaches the stomach. Individuals needing this medicine are often very thirsty for cold water.

child does not want to let go of her mother's hand. The medicine is *Bismuth*. People needing this medicine find solitude unbearable.

Hayley responded so well to the *Bismuth* that her mother did not bring her back for a year, at which time her symptoms had recently returned after she had eaten devil's food cake flavored with espresso. She became more content to play by herself. Hayley no longer grilled her mother constantly about where she was going nor ran down the driveway of their house begging her not to leave. Nor did her mother have to give her three hugs and three kisses before Hayley would let her out of her sight. Hayley had stopped begging her mother to pick her up and carry her when big dogs were around. The bedwetting had also improved dramatically until the cake episode. We repeated the *Bismuth* for Hayley at that time. Her mother called one week later to say that Hayley's symptoms had already begun to improve again.

"I Get Afraid Every Night of Being Kidnapped or of the House Catching on Fire"

Jillian, Hayley's ten-year-old sister, had fears of her own. She confided in us, "I get afraid at night. I've just lately been able to sleep in my own bed. My most fear is either one of us being kidnapped or a fire starting in our house. It happens every single night. I used to always go into my parents' room to sleep when I was really little. It was better until I was four and saw a television show about a fire." Her fear was even greater recently after some other kids started a fire near their house.

Whenever she and her family went to a shopping mall, Jillian stayed close to her parents so that no one could snatch her. She was concerned when her mother went out that she might get lost.

Jillian's mom described her as "a hysterical little girl." She woke up between midnight and two in the morning feeling unsafe. On those nights when her parents would not let her sleep on the floor of their room, she could not sleep all night. Jillian had to be careful about reading mystery books because they made her feel tense.

A whiz at learning, Jillian was a very fast reader with an excellent memory. Her mood was upbeat. She was always happy-go-lucky except when she was afraid at night. Jillian was helpful and very talkative. Like her sister Hayley and her father, she was also bursting with questions. She became very frustrated if she was unable to get out what she wanted to say. If she had something to say and others did not want to listen, she would yell it out anyway. "I have to let it out before I can relax."

She learned best when she did so through talking. It was a challenge for her to learn when she could not talk, especially when she was excited about something. At those times she would want to tell her whole story in detail and other family members would be anxious for her to get to the point. Jillian did not handle teasing well. She enjoyed being active, playing soccer, dancing, and crocheting. Jillian had few physical problems except for hangnails and a wart on her foot.

We considered Jillian's fears to be her most outstanding feature. It is very unusual, in our experience, for a child to be so afraid that she could not even go to sleep at night. As with Hayley, we did not find the best medicine for Jillian the first time. We tried *Arsenicum album*, the medicine that helped Annie, as well as *Calcarea carbonica* (Calcium carbonate), another medicine for people who are preoccupied with safety issues. Neither of these two medicines had the profound effect on Jillian's fears that we had hoped.

Then, based specifically on Jillian's extraordinary fear of their house catching fire, undoubtedly her most unusual symptom, we gave her *Cuprum aceticum* (copper acetate). As with Hayley, the beneficial effects of Jillian's medicine lasted for a year, until she ate the same espresso-flavored cake. Jillian's mother called to report that the second dose of *Cuprum aceticum* worked the same day it was given. Once again Jillian's fear of fire diminished and she was able to sleep soundly.

We Knew Something Was Wrong from the Moment He Was Born

Damien was a challenging little boy for his parents, his day-care providers, his previous homeopath (who had tried nine different medicines over the period of a year without success), and, not surprisingly, for us. Perhaps nine was the magic number for Damien, because it took that many trials for us, over a year and a half, to find the right medicine for him. Now, you might wonder why a parent would doggedly stick with homeopathy for so long, with two different physicians. The answer is simple: she was desperate, Damien was over the top, and nothing else had worked. It is a credit to his mom, Joyce's, patience and determination that we were able to help Damien. Here is his story.

"From the moment of birth, we knew something was wrong, but no one would listen. Damien cried all the time. It wasn't just how often he cried, but the tone of his wails. As if he were in pain. He never slept more than fifteen minutes at a time, then he'd wake shrieking.

Nursing him was rough because his body became rigid, he hated being touched, and he vomited constantly. When he nursed, he clawed at me, which really hurt." As his mother recounted her past trials with Damien, he dashed in and out of the office, chattered nonstop, and was into everything within his sight and reach.

Joyce continued, "My husband and I moved to a different state during the pregnancy. I was thrilled to be having him. I developed gestational diabetes at birth so he was in the neonatal intensive care for the first twenty-four hours, where he was bottle fed. During labor, they gave me Demerol and Tributaline to halt the premature contractions. Makes you feel like you're on speed. I couldn't keep enough food in him due to his continual vomiting, so I continued to give him a bottle to keep up his weight. Damien just kept screaming and screaming. I finally had him hospitalized at five months of age. They diagnosed him with reflux disease and a spastic ileocecal valve. He's never had a normal bowel movement—either constipation or diarrhea. They put him on lots of drugs. Damien didn't talk until he was almost two and a half. I had to teach him to crawl and walk. He continued to throw up to the point of projectile vomiting."

"My previous homeopath referred me to you. We also wondered about chemical sensitivities and tried an elimination diet. Damien is hyper and he never slows down or stops talking. He's perpetually fidgeting, has absolutely no impulse control, and he has frequent attacks of rage during which he attempts to hurt himself and others. Damien can be a sweetheart, but can also turn into a monster in a split second. That's when he lashes out to hurt whoever happens to be nearby or tears up his room. Once he's wound up, it's really difficult to calm him down."

"All of a sudden, Damien becomes extremely frightened. He acts like you or I might if someone held a gun to our head. In a flash, he's seized with panic. We can be sitting there quietly reading a book or he's eating breakfast, then, instantly, he becomes terrified and begins to scream out of control. When Damien's like that, thrashing about, there's no way to console him. Anything can scare him—his food, a shoe, his grandmother. It's a pity that he's never allowed her to get close to him because she adores him so. He can't tolerate any affection from her. He's equally afraid of his uncle."

Damien suffered from night terror a couple of nights a week. When he was younger, it was twice each night, and his mother was up with him regularly. Damien didn't know how to be gentle with animals. He could be petting them nicely for a minute or two then, all of a sudden, he'd yank on their ears, tails, or neck. His mother was struck by how irrational Damien's fears were. A chair could terrify him but he was not intimidated by the dark, animals, or water, as are many children.

It wasn't only Damien's fears and moods that were out of the ordinary. So were his physical symptoms. When we inquired about high fevers, his mom confirmed that unexplained fevers of 105 degrees Fahrenheit were commonplace. "Just a fever. No other symptoms. We called him 'toaster boy' the first year because he was hot all the time." Damien had experienced only one ear infection, a minor one at that. "He still gets fevers that come and go suddenly. Damien had surgery for a double hernia and hydrocele at five years."

Damien's rage was directed primarily towards his mother and himself. Pushing, hitting, hugging too hard. "Everything he does is too hard. He loves to be with other kids, but if the least little thing sets him off, he'll throw something at you and hit you smack in the head. It doesn't help that he's ambidextrous! This child goes wild. He can demolish a room in seconds. Sometimes I have to sit on him to get him under control." Exaggerated sensitivity to smell and light were also characteristics of Damien, as well as frequent stomach pain. He loved seafood and root beer.

We tried a number of medicines, including *Belladonna*, *Stramonium*, *Tuberculinum*, and *Veratrum album*, some of which produced up to a 40 percent improvement in his symptoms, but we were not satisfied. A year ago we changed the prescription to *Aconite* (Monkshood), a medicine for tremendous fright and fear of death as well as high fevers of sudden onset.

It was nine months before we heard again from Damien's mom. "That last dose—he was a different kid. Damien was actually hearing me when I talked to him. He wasn't hyper or chattering or fidgety. Damien went to the bathroom every day, had no stomach aches at all, and was eating much better. Even his skin was healthier. He did phenomenally well until he received his booster DPT shot at the end of November. A combative, aggressive episode like he used to experience occurred right after the immunization. Then the homeopathy kicked back in. Recently all of his old symptoms are coming back. Damien's throwing things around again, his grades have plummeted, and the aggression at school has returned. He's back to chattering again. The teachers and therapist are calling me to find out what's happened to him."

"I swear he was 90 percent better. Almost normal. A different kid. I could wash my hair while he was in the bedroom without his destroying the house. Damien was doing great getting along with other kids. Now he's mouthy and coming home with red marks on his head from running into walls or counters. Lately, before going to sleep, he runs through everything bad that can possibly happen. It's only after I tell him every detail of what will happen the next day that he can calm down and go to sleep. And that's after he's sure to remind me to turn out the lights and lock all the doors. His stomach aches are horrible again."

We repeated the *Aconite* in the same potency, but this time Damien was only 75 percent better overall. The teacher and therapist again noticed a marked improvement. Most of his symptoms were significantly better, but not as much as after the first dose. We gave him a higher dose of the medicine and again he has improved remarkably.

Fear, Negativity, and Rage Masquerading as Depression

We have found in nearly all cases of violent behavior in children and adolescents that beneath the bravado and rage lie fear and often terror. Homeopathy seeks to understand each child at the core; to address the underlying issues and perceptions rather than merely the superficial reactions. Of course, in a child who shrieks, insults, bites, kicks, and thrashes, the aggressive behavior is what stands out the most. But to find the homeopathic medicine that can literally transform a child's life, it is often necessary to probe more deeply. It is often only through engaging in one or more heart-to-heart conversations with the child or adolescent that the true emotions and motivations become evident.

This first case is an example of a child who would typically be diagnosed with oppositional-defiant disorder and depression. On examining the case further, however, fear is the crux of the problem.

Jeannie was ten. Her mother was a longtime patient of ours and knew that her daughter needed help. The family had moved from Seattle to Idaho a number of years previously. Jeannie's mother asked that we treat her daughter by telephone, which we did. Jeannie was very pretty with blond hair and blue eyes, but she was not at all happy with the way she looked.

Recently Jeannie complained that she hated life. Nothing pleased her. She talked of wanting to die and of killing herself. She threatened, "I'm gonna kill myself. I'm gonna take a knife and kill myself." When her distraught mother tried to talk to Jeannie about it, she would refuse.

Jeannie refused to do anything her mother or teacher asked of her. She seemed angry all the time, dissatisfied, and very argumentative. If anyone opposed her wishes, she snapped back and quarreled with them. Jeannie's mom described her as a perfectionist. If it weren't just right, she wouldn't do it. Trying to make her bed without any wrinkles just about drove her crazy.

During fits of rage Jeannie would slam doors until the house shook, throw the nearest object, hit, and scream, "I hate you. I want to leave." These episodes would come on very quickly. Even little disappointments threw her into a fury.

"I just don't like life," Jeannie told us. "It's everything. I don't like where we live. I don't like my teacher. I don't like our school." She did not like herself, felt jealous of her sister, and complained that her mother loved her sister more than her. Jeannie believed that she was unfairly treated all the time.

Jeannie had been very unhappy about the family's move to Idaho. She had a very hard time with friends. They were very important to her, but she did not have an easy time making friends. They told her that she whined too much and was not a good sport. She was exceptionally sensitive and became easily offended at the smallest things. Jeannie snapped back at her friends, insisting that she did not want to have anything to do with them. She worried constantly that people would not like her, and when she was mean to them, they did not. Jeannie was very embarrassed by the warts on her knees and kept them covered with Band-Aids.

Homeopaths often notice a correlation between the mental and emotional state of the mother during pregnancy and the state of the child later in life. When we inquired about the mother's pregnancy, she informed us that her husband had left her during her pregnancy with Jeannie. She felt a lot of sadness. There was a profound feeling of being unsupported. During this time they lost their house and all their possessions.

Jeannie was afraid of aliens, monsters, the dark, dead people, heights, and graveyards. She feared the dark because she thought monsters lived there, and deep swimming pools because there might be a shark lurking below the surface or an octopus that could grab her. Once she got a frightening thought into her head, she could not get it out. Jeannie also feared heights and remained glued to her mother when they hiked along steep areas. Jeannie also had nightmares of people chasing her and trying to kill her.

When we asked Jeannie's mother when all the fears began, she remembered one time when she woke up during a fever screaming, "They're gonna come get me." It was like a craze went through her. She clung to her mother very tightly during the fever. She was afraid to turn around to see the monster.

Jeannie's only physical problems now were headaches, rashes around her neck, and an intolerance for hot weather.

We were struck by the intensity of Jeannie's anger and her fears. They had a violent quality. She struck out with anger unpredictably, almost like something took over her. As with Peter and Kevin in the chapter on violence and rage, we gave Jeannie one dose of *Stramonium*. It is also known as a medicine for fright following a fever or a traumatic event.

We talked to her mother by phone five weeks later. Jeannie was doing much better after the first ten days. She was more in control of her emotions, and now could even talk about her feelings, which previously had seemed impossible. She was considerably less angry, bored, and dissatisfied. She was no longer jealous of her sister. Jeannie had expressed no more urges to kill herself.

Her sensitivity to criticism and her self-image had improved, but she still did not believe she was pretty or intelligent. Her light-heartedness was beginning to return. The day before the follow-up interview, she told her mother that she felt happier than she had in a long time. She still was afraid of heights, but now she would go down to the basement, previously an impossible goal. She received the medicine nearly a year ago and has been just fine since.

20

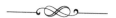

"I Feel Bad About Myself.
I Have No Friends."
Depressed Kids

The prevalence of depression during childhood varies greatly according to research studies, ranging from 1.9 to 13.9 percent. Depression seems more prevalent among children from special populations, such as children who are referred for learning problems.[6] The number of prescriptions of Prozac and Zoloft written for children aged five to ten were as high as 200,000 in 1994, reflecting a fourfold increase over a two-year period.[7] From 1991 to 1995, the number of preschoolers on antidepressants increased 200 percent.[8] As we mentioned earlier in this book, the number of children and adolescents, even toddlers, for whom Prozac and other antidepressants are being prescribed, frequently off label, is high

---

[6] Philip C. Kendall, ed., *Child and Adolescent Therapy, Cognitive-Behavioral Procedures* (New York: The Guilford Press, 1991), 171–172.

[7] G.J. Emslie, J.T. Walkup, S.R. Pliszka, and M. Ernst, "Non-tricyclic Antidepressants: Current Trends in Children and Adolescents." *Journal of the American Academy of Child and Adolescent Psychiatry* 38(5): 517 (1999).

[8] Karen Peterson and Kathy Kiely, "White House Seeks Study on Drugging of the Young." *The News Tribune*, March 21, 2000, A8.

enough to attract a study sponsored by the federal government.[9] Also discussed in the chapter on conventional medications for kids, one psychiatric newsletter compiled marketing data revealing that 2,000 prescriptions for Prozac alone were written for children under the age of one in 1994.[10]

Is life simply more overwhelming and depressing for children as young as three or four years of age? Is our awareness of "symptoms" so keen that we have changed the criteria for diagnosing depression in kids? Is our society more negative, malicious, and derogatory so as to drive even toddlers to depression? And, regardless of why so many children are being labeled with and medicated for depression, what are the other options for parents who don't choose to have their kids on psychotropic drugs, possibly for life? You, as a parent, undoubtedly want your child to be happy, self-confident, and socially accepted. Naturally, you want her to relate amicably to her peers and to enjoy the company of friends in and outside the school setting. A child with ADHD, or with other behavioral and learning issues, can find it challenging and frustrating to make and keep friends, attract invitations to birthday parties and sleepovers, and even to find company while eating lunch in the school cafeteria. Many of the kids we treat feel belittled, excluded, or ostracized by their peers. If a child continues to receive this type of treatment from his peers, he can become severely depressed during adolescence. The damage to self-esteem

[9] Ibid., A8.

[10] Julio Zito, Daniel Safer, Susan dosReis, James Gardner, Myde Boles, and Frances Lynch, "Trends in the Prescribing of Psychotropic Medications to Preschoolers." *Journal of the American Medical Association* 283(8): 1025 (2000).

and the ability to engage in healthy and loving relationships can even persist into adulthood.

You can see for yourself, in the following cases of children and adults suffering from depression and low self-esteem, how significantly homeopathic treatment can help.

"I Feel Like Someone Is Right Behind Me All the Time"

Natalie, age nine, could not keep up academically with the other children at school. She became easily distracted in a group setting, had difficulty concentrating, and found herself utterly lost when the other kids read too fast: "A long word struggles me," she explained. At all costs, Natalie wished to avoid revealing her problem understanding her teacher's requests. Instead, she became frustrated and angry.

Natalie also had a hard time getting along with her peers. They called her names, and she made faces back at them. Her facial tics made her the butt of their jokes. Feeling hurt and resentful, she, in turn, blamed the other kids for her troubles.

It felt to Natalie like someone was behind her, checking on her all the time. She even sensed someone following her during her sleep, which caused her to wake frequently. This nervous feeling of being watched haunted Natalie night and day. "I feel I have to run because someone is chasing me." Only when her mother stood behind her or snuggled against her did Natalie feel safe. She was particularly disturbed by a game she had played in which Mary Worth was behind her and Natalie had to stab Mary Worth.

Whenever Natalie's parents argued, she held herself responsible. They had divorced when she was three years old. A talker, Natalie had a tendency to chatter about things that didn't matter much. Though painfully aware that her behavior stood in the way of getting along with other kids, Natalie didn't know how to change it.

Natalie loved to bike, in-line skate, and draw. She hated smoking and would not tolerate it. She also had a strong aversion to guns, tobacco, and drinking. Natalie dreamed of horses and feared rattlesnakes because they could bite and poison her.

A warm-blooded child, Natalie's main physical problem was nosebleeds. They were quite severe, with clotted blood, and often lasted for fifteen minutes. She also had recurring mild hives.

Natalie was the first child we had ever met with such a strong fear of someone behind her in her waking state as well as in her dreams. This is an example of a case in which it was extremely important to understand the child's experience. Unfortunately many children tell us that they do not remember their dreams and do not share their fears as openly as Natalie. Her forthright approach to telling us her symptoms made it easier to prescribe for her.

We gave Natalie *Crotalus cascavella* (North American rattlesnake). Kids who need snake remedies often have interpersonal difficulties. They feel betrayed, abused, or attacked by others and often retaliate in a venomous way. This is manifested in a subtle manner by Natalie's resentment of other children who "get me into trouble." Animals in the wild are constantly threatened by predators and environmental dangers, so they need to be on guard all the time. Natalie manifested this type of vigilance. She checked all the time to see if someone were behind her, and she was always nervous that someone was watching her. She felt safe only with her mother behind her. She had trouble sleeping at night because she felt pursued. Natalie feared rattlesnakes "because they can bite and poison you."

People who need homeopathic rattlesnake can strike when threatened, often in a violent manner.

Natalie reported at her six-week follow-up visit, "The medicine really worked. I'm not calling people names. I'm not reacting. I'm not nervous." She no longer felt that someone was behind her and was now sleeping peacefully. Her reading, behavior in school, and overall performance had improved noticeably. Natalie's teachers were happy to report that she was more cooperative with her classmates and seemed eager to put her best foot forward. She had an increased desire to make friends. Her nosebleeds, cold sores, and hives were all gone.

When Natalie returned two months later, her physical complaints still had not returned. She had fewer problems at school. The feeling that someone was behind her had recently returned. She had a dream of a sea witch who was trying to take her brother away from their mother. In the dream, her mother had a glass of poison that she threw on the witch. Then her brother turned into a sea witch, too. The first witch had a potion that would make people die if

Crotalus cascavella (rattlesnake)

This medicine is made from rattlesnake venom. Children who need it feel that someone is behind them or hear footsteps following them. They have a characteristic fear of being alone and of ghosts and spirits and snakes. They can dream of hairy spiders. Intense, animated, hurried, restless, and talkative, they can suddenly strike out at others in a fit of rage. A characteristic physical symptom is hives, usually in one part of the body. Right-sided symptoms may be prominent.

it touched their hair. Natalie saved her mother and brother and the dream ended. The theme of poison even surfaced unconsciously in Natalie's dreams. We gave her another dose of the *Crotalus cascavella* because of the recurrent feeling of someone behind her.

At her visit seven months after the original dose of the medicine, Natalie was having no problems with the other children at school. She no longer worried that someone was behind her. Her mother described her as "a lot softer." School had not been a struggle since she began homeopathic treatment. She was still much more cooperative, and her dreams were no longer frightening. A year after beginning homeopathic treatment, Natalie continued to do well in all of these areas.

"Everybody Hates Me!"

Kimberly, six years old, was not happy with life. The family lived in Colorado, and we had already successfully treated her brother, by telephone consultation, for his terrible temper. Kimberly's mom hoped that we could help turn her daughter's life around for the better as well.

Kimberly's mother described her as "a wilted flower." She used to be fun and cute, but her personality had shifted dramatically. She became upset at the drop of a hat and threatened to run away or kill herself. She expressed the wish that she had never been born. Kimberly constantly complained that everyone hated her. She idolized her older sister, Mandy, who often mistreated her. When Mandy insisted on having her own bedroom instead of sharing, Kimberly made a bed for herself in the closet.

Kimberly's mother described her as inhibited. She was always afraid that people would laugh at her. She was too embarrassed to try out for cheerleading for fear she would not do it right the first time. Kimberly was crazy about gymnastics, but, if the teacher ever corrected her, she decided she did not like that teacher anymore. She hated to do anything wrong. If someone corrected her, she put her fingers in her mouth and wilted. She cried when accused of something or if her feelings were hurt. If someone rejected her or her mother reprimanded her, Kimberly would announce that she wanted to kill herself.

Clumsy and accident-prone, Kimberly would walk down the hall holding her baby brother and turn around so quickly that the baby's head would hit the wall. She felt remorseful afterward. She was uncouth and tactless. Kimberly had no comprehension of what was wrong with asking the disabled girl next door why she walked so funny or telling people to their faces that they were too fat. She made disparaging comments to her brother then passed them off as "just a joke."

Kimberly's mother described her as a "fire hydrant baby." She spit up her formula and the milk exited through her nose. A fun, sweet, bubbly baby and toddler, Kimberly earned the nickname of "Miss Social Butterfly." Now her temperament was the polar opposite.

Terrified of the dark, Kimberly was awakened often, especially by nightmares about people hurting each other or about scary creatures and monsters. Scary television shows also bothered her, and she insisted on being at her parents' side during thunderstorms.

What seemed most curious to us was Kimberly's personality shift. She went from being outgoing, fun, and life loving to being an unhappy, even miserable, child who often thought that she did not wan to continue living. A homeopath always seeks to understand what happened during a person's life at the time such a shift took place.

Sure enough, Kimberly's mother remembered one specific event that immediately preceded her personality shift. She had been on the playground when she was five years old and a little boy hit her in the head with a rock. Her mother had noticed the significant change at that time. Kimberly shared with us, "I thought I was asleep when he threw the rock at me. I used to remember how to write numbers, but after he hit me I sometimes forgot. Since that boy hit me with the rock, my mind just stops and I can't think clearly. Since that happened, it sometimes comes into my mind not to do nice things to people. I was never snotty before. When people are mean to me, I think I'm just a pile of trash. When the rock hit me, my mind just changed. If my brother or sister says something mean to me, I tell them I'm just gonna kill myself. I don't like living here."

There is a particular group of homeopathic medicines that are very helpful after a head injury, and one medicine that is most prominent for suicidal feelings after a head injury. It is *Natrum sulphuricum* (sodium sulphate), which also benefits people who feel scorned or criticized by friends or family members. Individuals needing this medicine are highly sensitive and can become very reclusive and despondent when they feel hurt or rejected. They take insults or perceived criticism so deeply to heart that they may even feel life is not worth living. Kimberly became so down on herself that she considered herself "trash" and became convinced that everyone hated her. It is shocking that a person can go from being so happy and outgoing to so depressed. We have, however, often seen this occur following head injuries.

We were relieved to hear from Kimberly's mother five weeks later that she was doing much better. She was considerably less accident-prone. She had substantially improved in her ability to stay on task and concentrate. She was no longer mean, and had stopped talking about wanting to die. She was much less sensitive. Kimberly reported, "I can remember stuff that I couldn't remember before like what I am going to do. My moods have been getting better. I haven't been getting very mad and I'm hardly ever crying anymore."

A call from her mother two months later revealed that Kimberly was still improving. Now able to act in a much more responsible way, she carried through on projects that she had not been able to complete before. Capable of staying on task without a chore list and following directions without becoming sidetracked, Kimberly was excited to tell her mother that she was making people laugh again like she used to do. Her mother described her now as "all-around pleasant," much more interested in learning. No longer depressed, Kimberly was able to take teasing much less to heart. She made no mention of wanting to die. Kimberly's mom remarked that she again had a bounce in her step and that her emotions had dramatically reversed since she started homeopathic treatment one year earlier.

"I'm Weird. There's Something Wrong with Me"

Candy was a strong-willed child, but very sensible and sweet. She was seven years old and had many of the same feelings that Kimberly had. Normally very obedient at school, now she began to have problems listening to her teacher's instructions and had to be reminded about the rules. Candy's mother found this very unchar-

Natrum sulphuricum (sodium sulphate)

This is a useful medicine for depression or other complaints following head injuries. The depression is primarily from being scorned in relationships or from despair about life. The child may feel very bad about himself, isolate himself, and may even consider suicide. The sadness is made worse with music. Children needing *Natrum sulphuricum* may be subdued or may have a wild side. They tend to experiment with drugs as teenagers. Physical manifestations of their problems include asthma and warts.

acteristic of her normally well-behaved child. Candy began to have a hard time following instructions at home, too. She told her mother that nobody liked her and she wished she were dead. "I'm feeling everyone around me is against me, even if they're my best friends. I can't trust people because they might hurt me. It makes me feel like no one really cares or likes me."

Her mother was also struck by Candy's outbursts of anger. "Sometimes I go to my room and slam the door, or I get mad. Inside I feel so alone. I get all burned up. It feels like someone's hitting you or like you have a pizza party for your friends and no one shows up. The boys tease me, and it really hurts . . . like you're falling and there's no one there to catch you. You fall flat on your face. It's like everyone's laughing at you and they're all your best friends. It makes me really sad. I feel like nobody likes me." Candy's teacher, on the other hand, told her mother that Candy had lots of friends at school.

Candy had a particularly upsetting time on Valentine's Day. She cried that she did not want to go to school and got in trouble that day, along with several other girls, for writing insulting valentines to several little boys. He mother had also found a family photograph with mustaches drawn over the faces. When she tried to talk with Candy about it, Candy replied, "Mom, I can't tell you." After much patience and listening on her mother's part, Candy finally told her that a boy at school had thrown dirt on her and called her a chicken. Most frightening to her was his threat to "mirtilize" her. She had even had dreams of running away from boys at school who were chasing her.

Over the next week, the situation at school deteriorated. Candy's mother got several frantic phone calls from the school, reporting that she was very upset and not getting along with her teachers. She felt sad and depressed and cried herself to sleep. She lamented to her mother, "My teacher doesn't like me and doesn't listen to me. My teacher told me that if I get another bad mark, then we'll need a parent conference. Mom, I'm a terrible person. Mommy, the sun's out and there's a big cloud in front of it. I just can't make the cloud go away." If homeopathy did not work quickly, Candy's mother planned to consult a child psychiatrist or psychologist.

Candy became progressively more defiant and would cry and cry if reprimanded, even for the smallest thing. She was adamant about not wanting to go to school. "I'm just gonna stay in bed and sleep. No one can hurt me if I stay asleep." She told her parents she hated them and threatened to never speak to them again. When upset, Candy sobbed and threw her stuffed animals on the floor. She became much sassier and her parents were afraid to say anything to her for fear of an exaggerated response. Candy's only physical problem was a tendency to redness and itching around the vagina and anus.

What exactly was Candy's problem? Why was it so hard for her to get along with her teacher and the other children and even her loving parents? We felt that she suffered from extreme over-sensitivity. She was very easily humiliated and the least reprimand made her feel that she was a very bad person. She was far too touchy and moody. We gave Candy *Colocynthis* (bitter cucumber), which is often needed by oversensitive, moody people. They become easily triggered by humiliation or hurt, and prefer solitude. They react with anger and indignation and can take everything the wrong way. It is typical for them to become defiant, pouty, and generally out of sorts.

We spoke by phone with Candy's mother six weeks later. She reported that Candy was able to handle herself without being too sensitive, and could take criticism much more easily. Her parents noticed a dramatic and positive shift in Candy's mood. Before, she had cried at the least problem and brooded for days. Now problems blew right over. Her red bottom was gone. She no longer had any problems at school. She was no longer defiant, although still strong-willed. Her mother explained,

Colocynthis (bitter cucumber)

Anger and indignation are the main feelings for people needing *Colocynthis*. These children are easily offended, especially by insults, humiliation, or feeling unappreciated. They are highly sensitive. Cramping pains, particularly in the abdomen, or sciatic pains in the legs are the most frequent physical problems. The pains are relieved by hard pressure or bending over.

"She's gonna do what she's gonna do. She thinks she's grown up." We found this to be quite normal.

Candy has continued to derive great benefit from *Colocynthis* over the four years since it was first given to her and has needed only three repetitions of the medicine.

"Life Is Like a Vacuum Cleaner. It Sucks."

Brian's mother brought him for help when he was sixteen. At the time of his first appointment, Brian initially denied having any problems. "Nothing at all is wrong. I don't have a life. I don't have freedom. I don't have anything. Life is like a vacuum cleaner. Even when it's really working, it sucks. I have no friends. There's nothing that I like to do and no one I can relate to." His mother felt that it was urgent for us to see him because, during a recent rage, he had tried to choke her.

Brian complained that his mother was controlling and blamed him for everything. He felt impulses to hurt her and other people. He found everything about his life depressing, worthless, and without value and doubted that he would ever by happy. Brian's teachers complained that he did not pay attention, but when they called on him in class, he always knew the answers. His teachers commented that Brian worked far beneath his potential.

Brian's mom described him as angry, depressed, and judgmental of others. His harsh language and manner was successfully building a wall between Brian and the world, to keep others at a safe distance. A very sensitive young man, in the past Brian had been witty, happier, and had loved telling jokes. Now he was miserable. It was as if he had an axe to grind against the world.

Brian revealed, "Most people hate me. I see no reason to love them. You get burned too many times. I quit trying a long time ago. I basically have nothing in common with the people I know. If I try to be nice, they treat me badly."

Brian fell on a sidewalk at age two and was once hit in the back of the head with a bottle. His parents divorced when he was four. He never found it easy to get along with other kids. He was always the one who got picked on. He still sometimes felt picked on and when he got really mad, he verbally attacked the nearest person. In third grade he threatened to throw himself in front of a car. In seventh grade he stood near a window and threatened to jump off the ledge. Brian reported having thought about committing suicide in junior-high school. He felt trapped, with nowhere to go.

We were very concerned about Brian. He was clearly depressed and very angry toward his mother. We gave her instructions to keep in close contact with us if there was any further violence. *Natrum sulphuricum* is the medicine we prescribed for Brian. It is the same medicine that we gave to Kimberly earlier in this chapter. It can benefit many people who have a nihilistic attitude toward life and severe, even suicidal, depression. They have often experienced scorn or criticism from others and, because of their sensitivity, can build a wall of protection to ward off feelings of vulnerability. These people often have some history of head injury.

We were relieved to hear two months later that Brian was doing much better. He had experienced no more violent outbursts, though he still got angry and screamed sometimes. There were no more fights at school. Brian had stopped feeling that he wanted to hurt his mother or someone else. He still felt that people hated him and that nothing gave him pleasure. When we asked Brian whether he would like to not feel depressed, he replied that he did not think that was possible. Brian complained that his tennis game was not as good now that he was not so filled with anger. Brian's mother remarked that his humor was starting to come back.

Five months after starting homeopathic treatment, Brian was working half-time at a grocery store and saving his money to buy a motorcycle. He admitted feeling better, but was unwilling to attribute the change to homeopathy, which he considered "a complete rip-off." He seemed to have some investment in believing that something his mother believed in could not help him. Brian admitted that he had no more suicidal thoughts. Homeopathy continued to be quite helpful to Brian, even if he did not think so. Unfortunately, due in part to his underlying nihilism and his anger toward his mother, he decided to discontinue treatment against her wishes. They have begun family counseling, which we hope will continue to move Brian in a positive direction. We have seen several cases where teenagers, despite being helped by homeopathy, unfortunately abandon treatment.

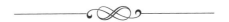

PART FIVE

Expanding Your Knowledge of Homeopathy

21

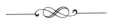

The Most Commonly Asked Questions About Homeopathic Treatment for ADHD

> ➤ *Can homeopathy help my child or me with ADHD?*

Most children and adults with ADHD can potentially benefit from homeopathic treatment; however, each case is individual. The cases in this book cover a wide range of behaviors and problems and provide a good idea of the scope of homeopathic practice. If you have specific questions, or if your own or your child's case is very complicated, call the homeopath first to make sure he or she feels that there is a good chance of homeopathy benefiting you. The more complicated the case, the more important it is to find an experienced practitioner.

> ➤ *Can homeopathy help my child with other problems?*

Homeopathy treats the whole child. Whether your child has ADHD, learning disabilities, asthma, allergies, or recurrent sore throats, there is a good chance that homeopathy can appreciably improve his or her health and well being.

➤ *My child's psychiatrist says his ADHD is caused by a biochemical imbalance. Can homeopathy help him?*

Homeopathy believes that any biochemical imbalance is a *result* of an overall imbalance in a person rather than the *cause* of ADHD. By bringing your child into balance as a whole person, you have the greatest chance of helping his behavioral, learning, and mood problems in a significant and lasting way. The goal of homeopathy is to bring about a profound improvement in your or your child's life and health, rather than only to regulate serotonin, dopamine, or some other neurotransmitter or chemical.

➤ *Ritalin helps my son's concentration for a few hours at a time, then he's bouncing off the walls more than before he took the medicine. Can homeopathy help?*

This is called "Ritalin rebound" and is a problem that many parents complain about. Homeopathic medicines last for months rather than only a few hours. Your child may experience an initial reaction to the homeopathic medicine lasting for a few days or, occasionally, two to three weeks, but then his behavior and academic skills should steadily improve. Since the doses are given very infrequently, this initial reaction is usually not much of a problem.

➤ *Stimulants seem to help my child pay attention, but they don't do anything for his self-esteem. Will the same be true of homeopathy?*

Definitely not. With successful homeopathic treatment, you should notice at least a 70 percent improvement in your child's academic performance, behavior, and self-confidence, as well as his ability to interact with others, to function in his life, and to be happy and healthy.

➤ *For how long will I have to continue homeopathic treatment?*

Most children need to continue under the care of a homeopath for at least two years. Significant progress is often noted within the first one to three months, as is evident in many of the cases that we have presented. Many families who are pleased with the results of their homeopathic treatment choose to use homeopathy for the rest of their lives.

➤ *How often will I need to see my homeopath?*

When first starting homeopathic treatment, visits are scheduled every six to eight weeks. After your child has responded well to treatment, your homeopath may only need to see him two to three times a year to help him stay as healthy as possible and prevent future illness.

➤ *How often will the homeopathic medicine be given?*

Homeopathic medicines may be given in single doses, in which case the medicine will only be repeated or changed when symptoms arise. As long as your child is responding well to the medicine he has taken there is no need to repeat it. If the improvement levels off or stops, or if the previous symptoms return, your homeopath will likely repeat a dose of the medicine. Homeopathic medicines may also be prescribed on a daily or weekly basis. If your child is taking a daily dose of homeopathic medicine, your homeopath may instruct him to continue taking the medicine for weeks or months.

➤ *What is the difference between taking a single homeopathic medicine and the combination homeopathic medicines that I have seen in my health food store?*

There is only one homeopathic medicine at any point in time that will have the most dramatic effect on your health. A trained and experienced homeopathic practitioner seeks to find that one specific medicine that most closely matches your symptoms. This exact or close match can produce profound and lasting healing. Combination medicines contain a variety of common homeopathic substances that have been found useful for such conditions as colds, flus, and sore throats. If the one medicine that you need is contained in that combination, you will respond well. If not, you will have no response or a partial response to the medicine.

Combination medicines should only be used for acute conditions when no qualified homeopath is available but should never be used for chronic or recurring conditions such as ADHD and the other conditions mentioned in this book. The same is true of chronic physical ailments such as asthma, headaches, eczema, and arthritis. For such conditions, find a trained, experienced homeopathic practitioner, and you or your child will have a much better chance of being helped significantly.

> *Are there side effects from homeopathic medicines?*

Homeopathic medicines are safe and gentle, yet they can produce powerful changes in people. There are no lists of side effects from particular homeopathic substances such as those from conventional medicines listed in the *Physician's Desk Reference* (PDR). There are certain symptoms that a person may experience as part of his or her healing process. These include an aggravation (brief flare-up of already existing symptoms within the first week of taking a homeopathic medicine) and a return of old symptoms (brief re-experiencing of symptoms that you have had in the past). Both an aggravation and a return of old symptoms are usually an indication that the medicine is a good match for you and will generally be followed by a significant improvement in your chief complaint and overall state of health. On rare occasions, an individual may experience a new symptom after taking a homeopathic medicine. If this happens, call your homeopath.

➤ *My child is taking Ritalin. Does he have to stop before beginning homeopathic treatment?*

No. Many of the children we treat are taking conventional medicines. We believe that it is best to find the appropriate homeopathic medicine first while continuing conventional drugs. Once your child is obviously doing much better, you can consult with the prescribing physician about decreasing or discontinuing the medicine. However, it is essential to tell your homeopath what your child is like when off all medications.

➤ *How long do I need to avoid the substances and influences that interfere with homeopathic treatment?*

It is advisable to avoid these influences as long as you are being treated homeopathically. There have been reports of symptoms returning after exposure to such influences up to two years after taking the homeopathic medicine. Some individuals, both children and adults, find that their treatment is *not* affected by coffee or other potentially contraindicated substances. At least wait until the correct homeopathic medicine has been prescribed. If it stops aching following an exposure to an antidoting substance or influence, your homeopath can repeat it. In some cases, when antidoting influences are unavoidable, a daily dose of the homeopathic medicine can be prescribed.

➤ *What if my child or I have food or environmental allergies?*

Homeopathy treats the whole person. When you or your child takes a homeopathic medicine that closely matches the symptoms and state, increased energy and vitality and a stronger immune system will follow. Often children who respond well to homeopathy can return to eating foods or being exposed to substances that bothered them prior to beginning homeopathic treatment.

➤ *I can't get my son to stop eating junk food. Will homeopathy still work for him?*

Although it is much healthier for children to eat fresh, whole foods and to avoid the empty calories found in high sugar, fat, and processed foods, the right homeopathic medicine will still be effective for junk-food addicts.

➤ *Your cases sound extreme. Can homeopathy work for more "normal" children?*

Homeopathy can be beneficial to many people. Those with very extreme, intense symptoms tend to need medicines made from more intense substances in nature, such as rattlesnake, scorpion, rabies, and tarantula. Other milder, more even-tempered people may need more gentle medicines such as those made from flowers.

➤ *How can I find a qualified homeopath in my area?*

See "Referral Sources for Homeopathic Practitioners" in the Appendix.

➤ *What if there is no experienced homeopath in my area?*

Some homeopaths are, as we are, willing to treat patients by phone or to do so after an initial in-person appointment. Telephone interviews are conducted just the same as if they occurred in person. We have found the results to be quite good. A local physician can perform any physical examinations that might be needed, especially for acute care.

➤ *How do I know if my local homeopath practices the same way that you describe in your book?*

Ask the practitioner if she practices classical homeopathy, uses one medicine at a time, and spends at least one hour with the patient during the initial interview. The answer to all of these questions should be yes. Ask where the practitioner was trained. It should be a course with a bare minimum of 500 hours, and, preferably, two years or more, in addition to ongoing seminars, conferences, and training. Find out how long the person has been practicing homeopathy and what percentage of his or her practice is homeopathy. Look for a homeopath who graduated from an accredited or well-respected program of training and who devotes a minimum of 75 percent of her practice to homeopathy. Board certification is optimal. Make sure that the practitioner is selecting medicines through an in-depth interview process rather than using machines, pendulums, or muscle testing to select the medicine.

➤ *Can homeopathic medicines made from toxic substances ever poison the people taking them?*

Never. Homeopathic medicines are diluted one part to nine or ninety-nine parts from six to one hundred thousand times. The medicines carry the pattern of the original substance but, if tested, would never contain enough of the substance to be toxic or dangerous. Arsenic, snake venom, strychnine, and rabies are all homeopathic medicines, but are absolutely nontoxic as homeopathic medicines.

➤ *How expensive is homeopathic treatment?*

The only significant expense for homeopathic treatment are the office visits, which last from one to two hours for the initial visit and approximately thirty minutes for follow-up visits. Cost depends on the experience, qualifications, and training of the practitioner. The cost of the homeopathic medicine itself is negligible. A year's worth of homeopathic medicine usually costs less than one prescription of many conventional medicines.

➤ *Are there insurance companies that cover homeopathic medicine?*

A minority of homeopathic practitioners is covered by insurance for a variety of reasons. First, many homeopaths are concerned about the issue of protecting their patients' confidentiality. Second, insurance companies rarely reimburse adequately for extended visits, such as the one-and-a-half hours to two hours necessary for an initial appointment. Third, many homeopaths are independent, progressive-type individuals who prefer the freedom of relating to patients apart from a managed-care or insurance-influenced system.

22

Our Society Needs
Homeopathy Now

We firmly believe that the over-medication of millions of children has gone way too far. We are not alone. In recent months, the dramatic increase in troubled children and the excessive use of Ritalin and other drugs to treat them has made front-page news. Influential people in positions of power have finally begun to respond. The American Academy of Pediatrics just issued its first guidelines for diagnosing ADHD, "hoping to prevent merely rambunctious youngsters from being overmedicated while ensuring other children get the help they need."[1] You may be surprised to learn this was not already the case—Ritalin has been prescribed for hyperactive children since 1955!

White House officials in the Clinton administration announced that the federal government will intensify research on medications used to treat preschoolers for behavioral problems, in response to growing concerns about the number of youngsters taking medications like Ritalin and Prozac. A five-year, $5-million research project has been funded to study children who take Ritalin for ADHD. The funds will also be used to redouble efforts to study labeling and dosage of psychiatric

[1] Lindsey Tanner, op. cit., A1.

drugs for youngsters and to convene a conference on the subject.

The Colorado Board of Education has passed a resolution discouraging teachers from making recommendations for medical evaluations of ADHD and treatment with Ritalin and encouraging them to find other means, instructional and disciplinary, to handle behavior problems in the classroom.[2] This step, we believe, sets an excellent precedent for putting diagnosis and treatment back into the hands of physicians, where it belongs, as well as further empowering parents and children.

We believe that we have found a far better way to manage ADHD than by treating millions of children with stimulant medication. Our aim is to help these children become all that they can be at level, to give them the best odds of turning into creative, loving, well-adjusted, productive, responsible, happy adults. As is evident from the many cases in our book, homeopathy works, plain and simple, and is very effective for many children and adults with ADHD. It is time for homeopathy to be recognized by the medical community, to be represented at the White House, to be brought into the awareness of physicians and educators. As you can see from this book, the scope of homeopathic medicine is vast, and its possibility to diminish suffering is tremendous. With this book, many more children and adults can learn about and benefit from this remarkable form of natural medicine.

The challenges and opportunities of our society and our planet are great. Ours is a rapidly changing and evolving world. We all seek happiness and well-being, yet we don't always know how or where to find

---

[2] Michael Janofsky, "Behavior Drugs for the Young Debated Anew," *New York Times*, November 25, 1999, 1.

it. The following words are attributed to a student from Columbine High School, Littleton, Colorado:

> The paradox of our time in history is that we have taller buildings but shorter tempers; wider freeways but narrower viewpoints; we spend more but enjoy it less. We have bigger houses and smaller families; more conveniences but less time; more degrees but less sense; more knowledge but less judgment; more experts but more problems; more medicine and less wellness. We have multiplied our possessions but reduced our values. We talk too much, love too seldom, and hate too often. We've learned how to make a living, but not a life . . . These are days of two incomes, but more divorce; of fancier houses but broken homes. It is a time when there is much in the show window and nothing in the stockroom; a time when technology can bring this letter to you and a time when you can choose either to make a difference . . . or just hit delete.[3]

Homeopathy is indeed a way to provide less medicine and more wellness—a way to truly make a difference. May more and more parents, educators, physicians, mental health professionals, legislators, and anyone who is in a position to help children, adults, or themselves learn about the wonderful benefits that homeopathy has to offer. And may millions of children reap the benefits.

[3] From an e-mail message forwarded to us on the Internet, "Powerful Words from a Student from Columbine High School", May 25, 2000.

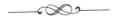

Appendix: Learning More

Recommended Books

Attention Deficit/Hyperactivity Disorder

Alexander-Roberts, Colleen. *AHDH and Teens: A Parents Guide to Making It Through the Tough Years.* Dallas: Taylor Publishing Company, 1995.

Barkley, Russell. *Attention Deficit Hyperactivity Disorder: A Handbook for Diagnosis and Treatment.* New York: Guilford, 1990.

DeGrandpre, Richard. *Ritalin Nation: Rapid-Fire Culture and the Transformation of Human Consciousness.* New York: W. W. Norton, 1999.

Diller, Lawrence. *Running on Ritalin: A Physician Reflects on Children, Society, and Performance in a Pill.* New York: Bantam Doubleday, 1998.

Garber, Stephen. *Beyond Ritalin: Facts About Medication and Other Strategies for Helping Children, Adolescents, and Adults with Attention Deficit Disorders.* New York: HarperCollins, 1997.

Hallowell, Edward M., and John J. Ratey. *Driven to Distraction.* New York: Simon and Schuster, 1994.

————. *Answers to Distraction.* New York: Pantheon, 1995.

Hartmann, Thom. *ADD Success Stories.* Grass Valley, CA: Underwood Books, 1995.

————. *Attention Deficit Disorder: A Different Perspective.* Novato, CA: Underwood-Miller, 1993.

Kelley, Kate, and Peggy Ramundo. *You Mean I'm Not Lazy, Stupid or Crazy?!* Cincinnati: Tyrell and Jerem, 1993.

Reichenberg-Ullman, Judyth, and Robert Ullman. *Rage-Free Kids: Homeopathic Treatment of Defiant, Aggressive, and Violent Children.* Rocklin, CA: Prima, 1999.

Wilens, Timothy. *Straight Talk About Psychiatric Medications for Kids.* New York: Guilford, 1998.

Homeopathy

Bellavite, Paolo, and Andrea Signorini. *Homeopathy: A Frontier in Medical Science.* Berkeley: North Atlantic, 1995.

Reichenberg-Ullman, Judyth, and Robert Ullman. *Prozac-Free: Homeopathic Medicine for Depression, Anxiety, and Other Mental and Emotional Problems.* Rocklin, CA: Prima, 1999.

————. *Rage-Free Kids: Homeopathic Treatment of Defiant, Aggressive, and Violent Children.* Rocklin, CA: Prima, 1999.

Ullman, Dana. *The Consumer's Guide to Homeopathic Medicine.* New York: Tarcher/Putnam, 1995.

————. *Discovering Homeopathy: Your Introduction to the Art and Science of Homeopathic Medicine.* Berkeley: North Atlantic, 1988, rev. ed. 1991.

Ullman, Robert, and Judyth Reichenberg-Ullman. *Homeopathic Self-care.* Rocklin, CA: Prima, 1997.

————. *The Patient's Guide to Homeopathic Medicine.* Edmonds, WA: Picnic Point Press, 1995.

Internet Homeopathic Resources

Web Sites of Judyth Reichenberg-Ullman, N.D., and Robert Ullman, N.D.

Main site:
www.healthyhomeopathy.com

Includes excerpts from all of our books, information for ordering books and kits and for scheduling appointments, our current conference and lecture schedule, and announcements about our upcoming books.

Secondary site:
www.healthy.net/jrru:

Includes more than one hundred articles by us on homeopathy and holistic healing, audiotapes on treating various acute and chronic conditions with homeopathy, excerpts from some of our books.

Special interest sites
  www.ritalinfreekids.com
  www.ragefreekids.com
  www.prozacfree.com
  www.wholewomanhomeopathy.com
  www.homeopathicselfcare.com

Homeopathy Home Page:
www.homeopathyhome.com/

A major homeopathic site with many links and resources.

National Center for Homeopathy:
www.homeopathic.org/

Newsletter, study groups and conferences for laypeople and professionals.

HealthWorld Online:
www.healthy.net
Comprehensive online service specializing in information about alternative medicine. Includes free medline, journal articles, book excerpts, and audiotapes.

Internet ADHD Resources

Three very good sites with many links on ADHD:

www.adders.org/

add.miningco.com/health/add/

www.oneaddplace.com/

Homeopathic Book Distributors

Homeopathic Educational Services
2124 Kittredge Street, #71-Q
Berkeley, CA 94704
Tel: (510) 649-0294
Orders only: (800) 359-9051
Web site: www.homeopathic.com

The Minimum Price
250 H Street
P.O. Box 2187
Blaine, WA 98231
Tel: (800) 663-8272

Referral Sources for Homeopathic Practitioners

Homeopathic practitioners vary widely regarding level of medical or psychiatric training and experience, licensing or certification, expertise, and style of practice. Not all of the practitioners in the following directories necessarily use the same methods we have described in this book or are qualified to treat patients with serious mental illness.

Homeopathic Academy of Naturopathic Physicians (HANP)
12132 S.E. Foster Place
Portland, OR 97266
Tel: (503) 761-3298
Fax: (503) 762-1929

Board-certified naturopathic physicians

The National Center for Homeopathy (NCH)
801 N. Fairfax, #306
Alexandria, VA 22314
Tel: (703) 548-7790
Fax: (703) 548-7792

Practitioners of various qualifications and experience, licensed and unlicensed

Council for Homeopathic Certification (CHC)
PO Box 460456
San Francisco, CA 94146
Tel: (415) 789-7677

Licensed and unlicensed (primarily) practitioners who have passed a certification examination

American Institute of Homeopathy (AIH)
10418 Whithead Street
Fairfax, VA 22030
Tel: (703) 246-9501

Board-certified M.D.s and D.O.s

North American Society of Homeopaths (NASH)
1122 East Pike Street, Suite 1122
Seattle, WA 98122
Tel: (206) 720-7000

Unlicensed professional homeopaths

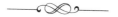

Glossary

acute illness—a condition that is self-limiting and short-lived, generally only lasting a few days to a couple of months.

Adderall—an amphetamine compound commonly used to treat ADHD.

aggravation—a temporary worsening of already existing symptoms after taking a homeopathic medicine.

allopathic medicine—a type of medicine, unlike homeopathy, which uses a different, rather than a similar, medicine to heal a set of symptoms

alternative medicine—natural approaches to healing that are nontoxic and safe, including homeopathy, naturopathic medicine, chiropractic, acupuncture, botanical medicine, and many other methods of healing.

amphetamine—a substance, whether prescription or recreational, that stimulates the nervous system; includes Ritalin, Cylert, Dexedrine, diet pills.

antidepressant—a substance that alleviates depression.

antidote—a substance or influence that interferes with homeopathic treatment.

antipsychotic—a prescription medication used to treat patients with schizophrenia and other thought disorders

Asperger's disorder—a high level of autism characterized by limited eye contact, peer relationships, and social interactiveness, as well as repetitive or stereotyped behaviors.

attention deficit disorder (ADD)—a diagnosis based on a constellation of symptoms that includes hyperactivity, attention problems, and/or impulsivity.

attention deficit/hyperactivity disorder (ADHD)—synonymous with ADD.

auditory integration—a method of integrating brain function and hearing that originated in France.

autism—a diagnostic category that includes withdrawal, introversion, difficulty with social interaction, ritualistic behaviors, and limited verbal communication.

case taking—the process of the in-depth homeopathic interview.

CH.A.D.D.—Children and Adults with ADD support group.

chief complaint—the main problem that causes a patient to visit a health-care practitioner.

classical homeopathy—a method of homeopathic prescribing in which only one medicine is given at a time based on the totality of the patient's symptoms.

combination medicine—a mixture containing more than one homeopathic medicine.

constitutional treatment—homeopathic treatment based on the whole person, involving an extensive interview and careful follow-up.

conventional medicine—mainstream Western medicine that follows orthodox views of diagnosis and treatment.

Cylert—a stimulant medication used for children with ADD.

defense mechanism—that aspect of the vital force whose purpose is to maintain health and defend the body against disease.

depression—a mood disorder characterized by persistent feelings of hopelessness accompanied by appetite changes, sleep problems, low energy or fatigue, and impaired self-esteem.

developmental disability—mental or physical delays in development and maturity due to genetic or congenital abnormalities; previously called mental retardation.

Dexedrine—a stimulant medication used for children with ADD.

DSM-IV—published by the American Psychological Association, the diagnostic and statistical manual that classifies mental and emotional disorders into diagnostic categories.

disruptive behavior disorder—a group of diagnoses manifested by behavioral patterns that are disruptive to others including attention deficit/hyperactivity disorder, oppositional-defiant disorder, and conduct disorder.

FDA—United States Food and Drug Administration.

Feingold diet—a dietary approach to treating ADD that includes the elimination of food colorings, additives, preservatives, flavorings, and salicylates.

gifted children—children classified with above-normal intelligence and learning abilities.

high potency remedies—remedies of a 200C potency or higher.

homeopathic medicine—a medicine that acts according to the principles of homeopathy.

homeopathic practitioner—an individual who treats people with homeopathic medicines according to the philosophy of homeopathy.

homeopathy—the use of a substance that causes a particular set of symptoms in a healthy person to relieve similar symptoms in a person who is ill.

Law of Similars—the concept that like cures like.

learning disability (LD)—difficulties with reading, mathematics, written expression, or other areas of learning

low potency remedies—remedies of a 30C potency or lower.

materia medica—a book that includes individual homeopathic remedies and their indications.

miasm—an inherited or acquired layer of predisposition.

minimum dose—the least quantity of a medicine that produces a change in the patient.

modality—those factors that make a particular symptom better or worse.

naturopathic physician—a physician who has graduated from a four-year naturopathic medical school and who treats the whole person based on the principle of the healing power of nature.

neurotransmitter—a chemical substance, like serotonin or dopamine, that transmits nerve impulses in the brain and nervous system, affecting thinking, behavior, sensory, and motor function.

nosodes—homeopathic medicines made from the products of disease.

obsessive-compulsive disorder (OCD)—a diagnostic category that includes symptoms of obsessive thought patterns and ritualistic behaviors.

oppositional-defiant disorder (ODD)—a pattern of negative and defiant behavior involving argumentativeness, resentment, vindictiveness, and abdication of personal responsibility

pervasive developmental disorder—a spectrum of diagnoses including autism, childhood disintegrative disorder, and Asperger's disorder.

phobia—an unreasonable, disproportionate, persistent fear of a specific thing.

potency—the strength of a homeopathic medicine as determined by the number of serial dilutions and succussions.

potentization—the preparation of a homeopathic medicine through the process of serial dilution and succussion.

prover—a person who takes a specific homeopathic substance as part of a specially designed homeopathic experiment to test the action of medicines.

provings—the process of testing out homeopathic substances in a prescribed way in order to understand their potential curative action on patients.

relapse—the return of symptoms when a homeopathic medicine is no longer acting.

remedy—a homeopathic medicine prescribed according to the Law of Similars.

repertory—a book that lists symptoms and the medicines known to have produced such symptoms in healthy provers.

return of old symptoms—the re-experiencing of symptoms from the past, after taking a homeopathic medicine, as part of the healing process.

Ritalin—a stimulant medication commonly used for ADD.

S.A.D.—School Avoidance Disorder (in other books this is also used as an abbreviation for seasonal affective disorder).

school refusal behavior—the refusal on the part of a child to go to school, usually associated with some type of fear.

serotonin—a neurotransmitter in the brain which can affect moods and behavior.

simillimum—the one medicine that most clearly matches the symptoms of the patient and that produces the greatest benefit.

single medicine—one single homeopathic medicine given at a time.

SSRI—one of a family of antidepressants that are selective serotonin reuptake inhibitors and, therefore, increase levels of serotonin in the brain

state—an individual's stance in life; how he or she approaches the world.

stimulant—a substance, prescription or recreational, which stimulates the nervous system.

succussion—the systematic and repeated shaking of a homeopathic medicine after each serial dilution.

symptom picture—a constellation of all of the mental, emotional, and physical symptoms that an individual patient experiences.

tic disorder—a symptom picture characterized by twitches, jerks, and other convulsive or uncontrollable behaviors.

totality—a comprehensive picture of the whole person: physical, mental, and emotional.

Tourette's disorder—a specific type of tic disorder that includes jerking, throat clearing, swearing, and other uncontrollable nervous system behaviors.

vital force—the invisible energy present in all living things that creates harmony, balance, and health.

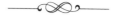

Index

Absentmindedness, 20, 132–136
Accident-prone behavior, 12
Aconite, for rage and phobias, 245–246
ADD. *See* Attention deficit disorder; Attention deficit hyperactivity disorder
Adderall, 44–49
ADHD. *See* Attention deficit hyperactivity disorder.
Adolescents, ADHD symptoms, 17–19
Adults with ADHD: behavior and symptoms, 19–21, 46; case studies, 188–205
Agaricus muscaria, for adult ADHD, 198–199
Alcohol abuse, 18
Allergies, homeopathic medicine for, 152, 271–272
Alternative medicine, 58–59
American Academy of Pediatrics, 275
Amitriptyline, 51
Androctonos, 178
Anger, 18
Angustura, 173
Animal cruelty, 12, 14
Antidepressants, short-term effects, 52
Antihypertensive drugs, 56–57
Antipsychotic drugs, 57–58
Anxiety, treatments for children with, 230–249
Appetite loss, Ritalin side effect, 45, 49
Arsenic, 236
Arsenicum album: for anxiety and phobias, 235–237; for phobic children, 241–242

Asperger's disorder, 212–215
Attention deficit disorder, 129–143
Attention deficit hyperactive disorder (ADHD): adolescents, 17–19, 117–119, 145–152; adults, 19–21, 46, 188–205; case studies, xxi–xxii, 117–187; children with, 1–17, 34–38, 108–114; common features, 3–21; diagnosis of, xviii; dietary factors, 27–29; drug treatments, pros/cons, 41–59; epidemic vs. overdiagnosis, 22–32, 38–40; family/environmental factors, 25–26; genetic factors, 25–26; gifted children and, 30–31; grade-schoolers, 14–17, 122–143; homeopathic treatments and effects, xx–xxi, 71–83; impulsive behavior, 7; infants, 11–12, 119–122; intelligence, 7–8, 21; manifestations, xiii; nature vs. nurture, 25–26; overdiagnosis by teachers, 29–30; overstimulating social environments, 26–27; parents with, 114; positive characteristics, 9; predisposition toward, 31–32; preschoolers, 12–14; restlessness, 6; Ritalin vs. homeopathic treatments, 82–94; selecting homeopath for, 93–94; underachievers, 7–8; urgency felt by children and caregivers, 33–39; violent behavior, case studies/treatment for, 166–187. *See also* Children with ADHD
Attention-seeking behavior, 16
Autism, 215–200

Barium carbonate, 225
Barium sulphate, 214
Baryta carbonica, for developmentally disabled, 225
Baryta sulphuricum, 214
Behavior, ADHD: adolescents, 17–19; adults, 19–21; gradeschoolers, 14–17; infants, 11–12; preschoolers, 12–14
Belladonna, for hostile behavior, 181–182, 245
Benzodiazepines, 56–57
Bipolar disorder, 53–55
Bismuth, 239–240
Bismuthum subnitucum, for anxiety, 239–240
Bitter cucumber, 261–262
Black hellebore, 118–119, 135–136, 174, 196, 220
Bufo rana, treatment for developmentally disabled, 223–226
Buspar, 56–57

Caffeine, ADHD and, 27
Calcarea carbonica, 135; for phobic children, 241–242
Calcarea phosphorica, 142; for oppositional-defiant disorder, 161–162
Calcium carbonate, 241–242
Calcium phosphate, 142, 161–162
Capsicum, for oppositional-defiant disorder, 157–158
Carcinosin, 142–143
Career, ADHD effects on, 19
Catapres, 56–57
Celexa, 52–53
CHADD (Children and Adults with ADD), 40
Children: anxieties and phobias, homeopathic treatments for, 230–249; behavior, 11–17; case studies, 34–36; crack cocaine, homeopathic treatments for, 226–229; depressed, homeopathic treatments for, 250–264; frustrations felt by, 33–39; gifted, 30–31; learning and developmental disabilities, 209–229; relationships with siblings and peers, 14, 16
Children with ADHD: appreciation for, 108–110; communicating with, 111–112; importance of consistency, 110–111; importance of limits, 110–111; nonstimulating activities for, 111–112; one task at a time, 110; parents' needs, 112–114; symptoms, 10–19
China, 212
Chocolate, as homeopathic treatment, 138–139
Cina, treatment for oppositional-defiant disorder, 159–160
Cinchona bark, 212
Clomipramine, 51
Clonidine, 43–44, 56–57
Clowning behavior, 16
Club moss, 131–132
Colocynthis, for anger and depression, 261–262
Colorado Board of Education, 276
Columbine High School, Littleton, Colorado, 277
Combative behavior, homeopathic treatments for, 173–175
Computer games, role in ADHD, 27
Concentration difficulties, 20
Conduct disorder, 168
Conventional medicine, homeopathy and, differences, 77–78, 83–86
Convulsive behavior, homeopathic treatment for, 226–229
Copper acetate, 242
Crack baby, homeopathic treatment for, 226–229
Criminal behavior, 167–168
Crohn's disease, 212
Crotalus cascavella: for adult ADHD, 202–203; treatment for depression, 253–255
Cucumber, bitter, 261–262
Cuprum aceticum, for phobic children, 242
Cylert, 44, 146

Datura stramonium, 170
Daydreaming, 15, 20
Defiant behavior, 13, 17–18; case studies, 153–165
Depakote, effects/side effects, 54–55
Department of Education, 43

Depression, 18; homeopathic treatments for, 250–264
Desipramine, 51
Desoxyn, 44
Destructive behavior, 13, 18
Desyrel, 52–53
Developmental disabilities, homeopathic treatments for, 209–229
Dexedrine, 44–49; autism and, 217
Dextroamphetamine. *See* Dexedrine
Diet, 27–29
Distracted behavior, 13
Dopamine imbalance, 24–25
Drug abuse, 18
Drug Enforcement Agency, xvii, 42
Drug treatments: case studies, 60–66; children's reactions, 60–66; medical researchers' opinions, 66–67; parents' opinions, 60–66; pros/cons, 41–59
Dyslexia, 212

Effexor, 52–53
Ephedra, 27
Epidemic, ADHD, 22–32, 38–40
Erythromycin, 53
Eye contact, poor, 10

Fast-food, role in ADHD, 28
Fidgeting, 16
Financial costs, of homeopathic treatments, 273–274
Fluoxetine, 50
Food and Drug Administration (FDA), 79–80
Frustration, as felt by ADHD children, 33–39

Gabitril, 55
Germanium, 212
Gifted children, ADHD and, 30–31
Grades, at school, 15, 17–18
Gratification, immediate, need for, 21
Growth retardation, short-term, as medication side effect, 49
Guanfacine, 56–57

Haldol, 57
Haloperidol, 57
Head injuries, homeopathic treatment for, 257–258
Helium, for autism, 218–220
Helleborus, 135–136, 220

Histaminum, for allergies, 152
Homeopathic Pharmacopoeia of the United States, 79–80
Homeopathic treatments, xx–xxi, 41–59; allergies and, 271–272; for anxiety and phobias, 230–249; for autism, 215–220; case studies, 86–89, 101–107; costs, 273–274; for defiant behavior, 153–165; for depression, 250–264; FAQs, 267–274; frequency of, 269; insurance, 274; junk food and, 272; for learning disabled and developmentally disabled, 209–229; length of, 269; natural substances as sources of, 78–79; for oppositional-defiant disorder, 153–165; side effects, 270–271; substances to avoid during, 90
Homeopaths: referral sources, 282–283; search for, 93–94, 273
Homeopathy, 71–81; ADHD case studies, 117–187; adolescent case studies, 117–119, 145–152; controversies behind, 76–77; conventional medicine and, differences, 77–78, 83–84; with conventional treatments, 85–86; as effective ADHD treatment, 82–94; grade-schooler case studies, 122–143; as health care in other nations, 80–81; infant case study, 119–122; Internet resources, 281–282; limitations, 91–92; model personalities, 97–100; physician opposition to, 89–90; regulation by FDA, 79–80; research studies, 74–76; self-treatments, 92; uniqueness of each treatment, 95–100. *See also* Homeopathic treatments
Hostile behavior, homeopathic treatment for, 181–182

Imipramine, 51
Immediate gratification, need for, 21
Impaired children, severely, 209–229
Impulsive behavior, 7, 12
Infants: ADHD symptoms, 11–12; behavior, 11–12
Injury, head, homeopathic treatment for, 257–258

Insomnia, as Ritalin side effect, 45, 49
Insurance, homeopathic treatments and, 274
Intelligence and ADHD, 7–8, 21
Internet, homeopathic Web sites on, 281–282
Interruptive behavior, 16

Job difficulties, 18–19
Junk food, homeopathic treatments and, 272

Kali bromatum, 125
Klonopin, 56–57

Lamictal, 55
Law of Similars, 71–72
Learning difficulties, 20
Learning disabilities, homeopathic treatments for, 209–229
Lithium, child case study, 162–165
Lithium carbonate, effects/side effects, 54–55
Luvox, 52–53
Lycopodium, 131–132
Lyssin, for violent behavior, 185–187

Manic-depression, 53–55
Medications, pros/cons, 41–59
Medorrhinum, as treatment for adult ADHD, 192–194
Mellararil, 57
Memory, ADHD effects, 20
Merrow Report, xvii, 22, 41, 66
Methylphenidate, usage, 39–40.
   See also Ritalin
Monkshood, 245–246
Mood stabilizers, effects/side effects, 53–55

National Institutes of Mental Health, 43
Natrum muriaticum, 127–128
Natrum sulphuricum: for suicidal feelings, depression, and head injury, 257–260; for violent behavior, 263–264
Natural substances, for homeopathic treatments, 78–79
Navane, 57
Neurontin, effects/side effects, 54–55

Neurotransmitter, abnormalities, 24–25
Nosode, 142–143, 193
Novartis drug manufacturer, 40

Obsessive-compulsive disorder, 53
"Off-label" dispensing of drugs, xix
Oppositional-defiant disorder, case studies, 153–165
Overdiagnosis: ADHD, 22–32, 38–40; role of teachers, 29–30

Parents: with ADHD, 114; of ADHD children, 112–114; in case studies, 37–38
Paxil, 52–53
Pediatrician, in case study, 38
Pediatrics study, 38–39
Personality types for children, based on animals, plants, and minerals, 97–100
Phobias, homeopathic treatments for, 230–249
Physical coordination, 16
Plantago, for adult ADHD, 204–205
Plantain, 204–205
Potassium bromate, 124–125
Potentization, 73
Predisposition toward ADHD, 31–32
Preschoolers, behavior, 12–14
Prescription drugs: case studies, 60–66; children's reactions, 60–66; medical researchers' opinions, 66–67; parents' opinions, 60–66; pros/cons, 41–59
Provers, 79
Provings, 78–79
Prozac, 43, 50–53, 52–53, 250–251; case studies, 60–66; child case study, 162–165; children's reactions, 60–66; medical researchers' opinions, 66–67; parents' opinions, 60–66
Psychiatric drugs for children, alternatives to, 58–59
Psychotropic medications, 41–59
Pulsatilla, for anxiety, 238–239

Rabies nosode, 185
Rage, case studies/treatment for, 166–187
Rattlesnake, 202–203, 253–255
Reading skills, 15, 20

Rebelliousness, 18
Red pepper, 157–158
Repetitive movements, 16
Restlessness, 6, 10
Risperidal, 57
Ritalin, xviii, 146; alternatives to,
    x; autism and, 216; case studies,
    60–66; children's reactions,
    60–66; excessive use, 275–276;
    homeopathic treatments and,
    comparison, 82–94; medical re-
    searchers' opinions, 66–67; par-
    ents' opinions, 60–66; pros/cons,
    41–59; as street drug, 49; usage,
    39–40
"Ritalin rebound," 268
Royal London Homeopathic
    Hospital, 80

Scorpion, for malicious behavior,
    177–178
Self-esteem, low, 18–20
Self-treatment, homeopathic, 92
Seraquel, 57
Serotonin, imbalance, 24–25
Sertraline, 50
Serzone, 52–53
Side effects, homeopathic, 270–271
Sleeplessness, 10, 12
Social skills, 20; underdevel-
    oped, 19
Society of Homeopaths, 80
Sodium chloride, 127–128
Sodium sulphate, 257–260
SSRI antidepressants, 50–53
Stelazine, 57
Stimulant medications for ADHD,
    xvii–xviii, 39–40, 45–46, 49;
    downside of, 48; increased usage
    for children, xvii–xviii; "off-
    label" dispensing of, xixi;
    pros/cons, 41–59; side effects, 49
Stimulation, need for constant, 11,
    19, 21
Stramonium, 245; for anger and
    fright, 249; for violent behavior,
    169–171, 176–177
Study abilities, 15, 17–18
Succussion, 73
Sugar intake, 27–28
Suicidal feelings, homeopathic
    treatment for, 257–258
Sulphur, 214; for autism, 220; for
    combative behavior, 173–175; as

homeopathic medicine, 87; for
    oppositional-defiant disorder,
    164–165

Tantrums, 12–13
Tarentula, 88–89, 121–123,
    146–148
Tavist, 53
Teacher complaints, 14, 16–17
Teachers: in case studies, 36–37;
    and ADHD overdiagnosis, 29–30
Tegretol, effects/side effects, 54–55
Television, role in ADHD, 27
Tenex, 56–57
Test-taking difficulties, 15, 17–18
Thioridazine, 57
Thiothixene, 57
Thorn apple, 170
Tirelessness, 12
Topamax, effects/side effects, 54–55
Tourette's disorder, 290; as medica-
    tion side effect, 49
Tricyclic antidepressants, 44, 50–53
Trifluoperazine, 57
Truancy, 17–18
Tuberculinum, 245
Tungsten, 173

Underachievers, 7–8

Veratrum album, 118–119, 245; for
    adult ADHD, 196; for combative
    behavior, 173; for developmen-
    tally disabled, 222–223
Violent behavior, 13; case studies,
    166–187; homeopathic treatment
    for, 185–187, 263–264
Vital force, 290

Web sites, 281–282
Weight loss, as medication side
    effect, 49
Wellbutrin, 52–53
Windflower, 238–239
Work, ADHD effects on, 19
Wormseed, 159–160

Xanax, 56–57

Zinc, 228–229
Zincum metallicum, for convulsive
    crack-cocaine child, 228–229
Zoloft, 50, 52–53, 250–251
Zyprexa, 57

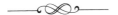

About the Authors

Judyth Reichenberg-Ullman, ND, DHANP, MSW, and Robert Ullman, ND, DHANP, are licensed naturopathic physicians and board-certified diplomates of the Homeopathic Academy of Naturopathic Physicians. Dr. Reichenberg-Ullman received a doctorate in naturopathic medicine from Bastyr University in 1983 and a master's in psychiatric social work from the University of Washington in 1976. Dr. Ullman received his naturopathic medical degree from the National College of Naturopathic Medicine in 1981 and completed graduate coursework in psychology at Bucknell University in 1975. Both had extensive experience in conventional mental health prior to their homeopathic training. The doctors practice at The Northwest Center for Homeopathic Medicine in Edmonds and Langley, Washington, where they specialize in homeopathic family medicine. For in-person or telephone consultations, call 425-774-5599.

Past president and vice president of the International Foundation for Homeopathy and past faculty members of Bastyr University, they teach, write, and lecture widely. They are frequent guests on radio shows across the United States, including *Talk of the Nation* and *The Voice of America*. They are authors of more than 250 articles and have been columnists for the *Townsend Letter for Doctors and Patients* since 1990.

Drs. Reichenberg-Ullman and Ullman are coauthors of *Rage-Free Kids, Prozac-Free, Homeopathic Self-Care,* and *The Patient's Guide to Homeopathic Medicine*. Dr. Reichenberg-Ullman is also the author of *Whole Woman Homeopathy*. You can order their books through their Web site at www.healthyhomeopathy.com or from Picnic Point Press, 131 3rd Ave. N., Edmonds, WA 98020 (800-398-1151), if they are not on the shelf of your local bookstore.

For More Information
Please visit our Web site,
RitalinFreeKids.com

From the Web Site:

We want to welcome you and let you know that we are here to help you and your family find an effective solution for ADHD. In our seventeen years of homeopathic practice, we have treated over two thousand people with ADHD, Oppositional Defiant Disorder, Learning Disabilities, Pervasive Developmental Delay, and other behavior and learning problems.

As a parent, relative, teacher, or counselor of someone with ADHD, or if you have ADHD yourself, you want to know what really works. You may have already tried conventional drugs, supplements, biofeedback, allergy testing, psychotherapy, or behavior modification. If you are tired of side effects and approaches that haven't worked for you, and you are seeking a safe, effective, non-drug alternative, you are in the right place.

What you will find there:

Our articles
Audio interviews
Our homeopathic books and kits
Sample chapters from our books
Our teaching and travelling schedule
Links to our other sites and sites on homeopathy or ADHD

Please visit our other sites, too:

RageFreeKids.com
WholeWomanHomeopathy.com
HealthyHomeopathy.com
ProzacFree.com
HomeopathicSelfCare.com